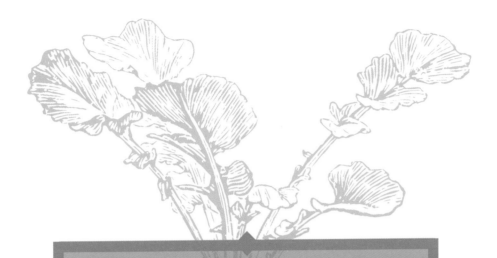

THE
DAILY VEGAN
A GUIDED JOURNAL

If found, please return to: _____

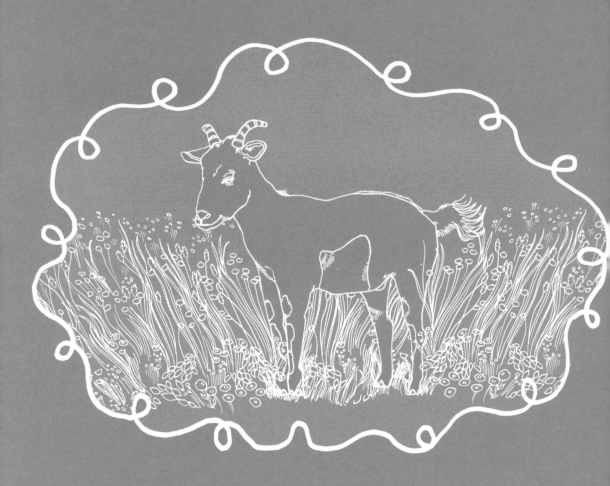

HOW TO USE THIS JOURNAL

Being vegan is more than a dietary choice—it's a philosophy of living, based on consciousness and compassion. [It's about doing the best we can to not contribute to the suffering of animals (human and non-human) we have the power to do so.]

Being vegan isn't about trying to attain an impossible level of purity or striving to be a 100-percent-certified vegan—the world is just too imperfect for that. It's about making daily choices in our lives and at our tables that reflect our deepest values. My hope is that this journal will be a guide for you as you venture and reflect on your own journey.

— Colleen Patrick Goudreau

SPEAKING YOUR TRUTH

Have you ever shied away from talking about being vegan to "protect" other people from discomfort? Think about it another way: By staying quiet, could you be denying other people the opportunity for the transformation that comes with honest communication?

Definitely.
　　Obviously, sometimes it would be inappropriate to bring it up, but I have definitely avoided using the V- word before

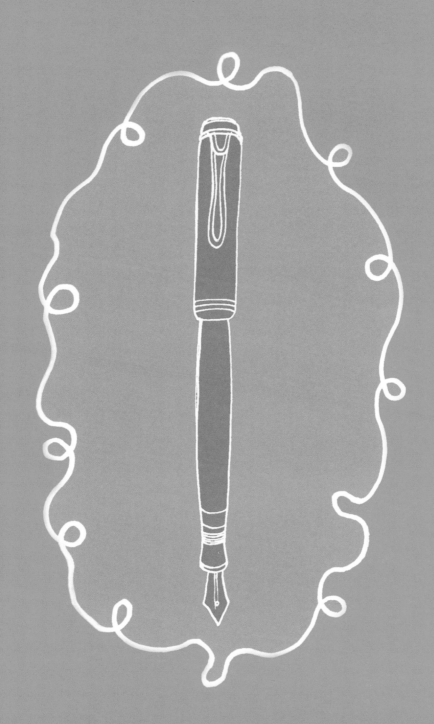

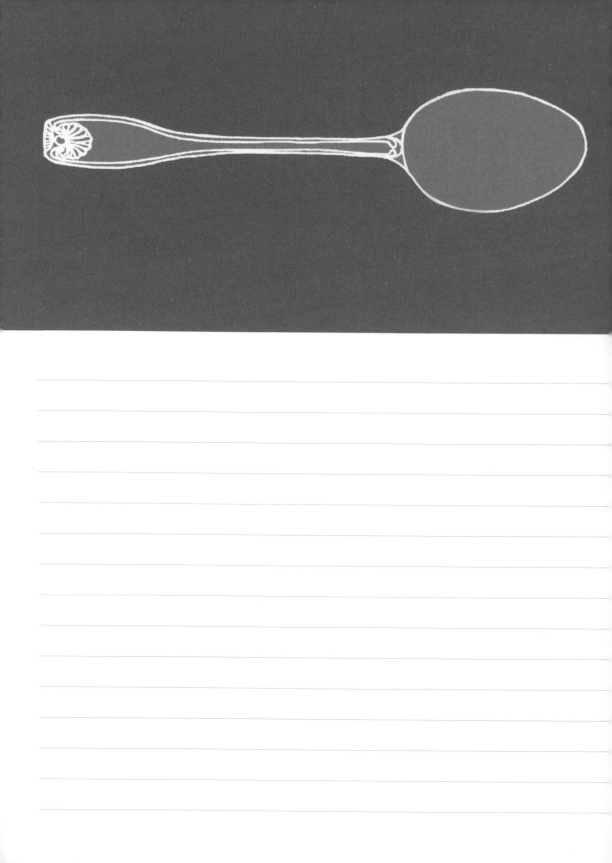

LENTILS

Lentils, part of the legume family, should be a pantry staple. They come in a variety of colors and textures and take no time to cook. Soft brown or red lentils are great for making patties, loaves and dal. Firmer green or black lentils are ideal for lentil salads. A cooking tip: Add salt when the lentils are nearly finished cooking. Salting earlier can slow the cooking process.

The heart is hard in nature, and unfit

For human fellowship, as being void

Of sympathy, and therefore dead alike

To love and friendship both, that is not pleased

With sight of animals enjoying life,

Nor feels their happiness augment his own.

— From "A Winter Walk at Noon" by William Cowper

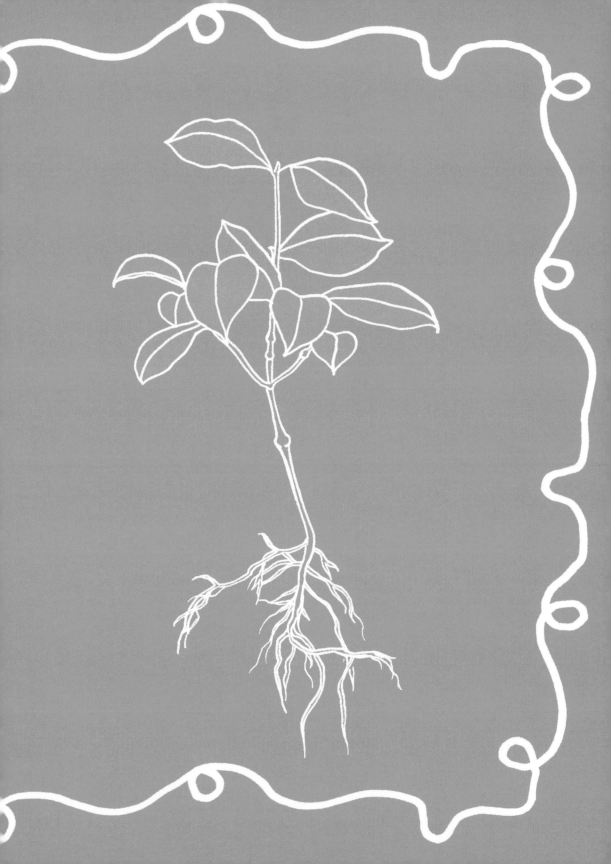

Notes

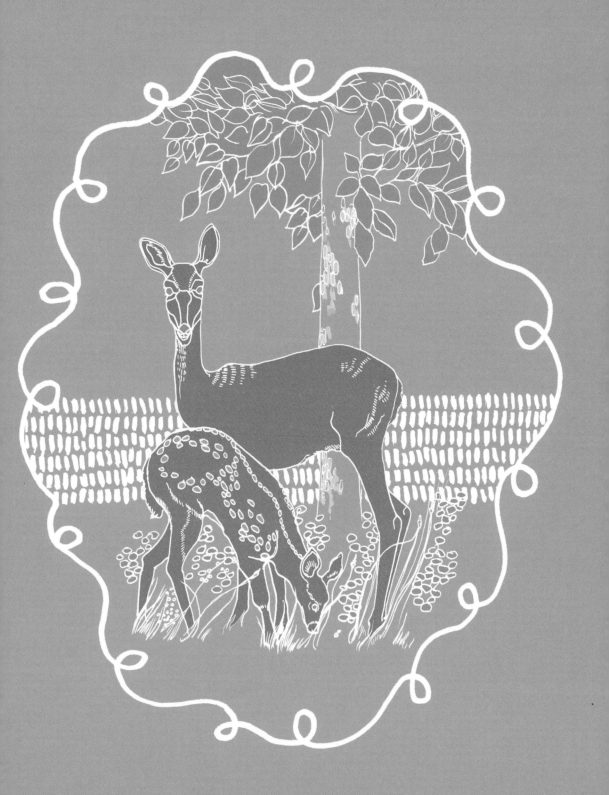

EATING MINDFULLY

Do you treat eating as a secondary activity, something to be done while driving, working, or watching TV? What would happen if you slowed down and thought of eating as a sensual experience where your senses of sight, hearing, taste, touch, and smell each played a role?

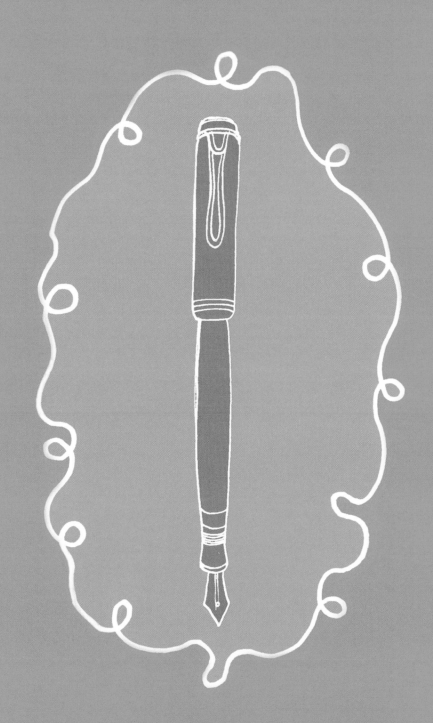

KALE

Kale is one of the most nutrient-dense foods on the planet. Some ideas for your daily dose of kale:

→ Sauté kale with garlic, olive oil, and salt. Add a little lemon juice before serving.

→ Massage raw kale for a few minutes to tenderize it and remove its bitter edge.

→ Add chopped kale to any soup or stew.

→ Blend kale into any fruit smoothie, or make a kale-centric smoothie with frozen bananas and apple juice.

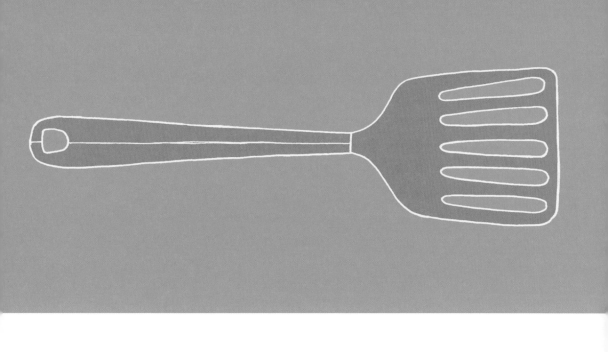

The wild deer, wandering here and there,
Keeps the human soul from care;

The lamb misus'd breeds public strife,
And yet forgives the butcher's knife;

Kill not the moth nor butterfly,
For last judgment draweth nigh.

The beggar's dog and widow's cat,
Feed them & though wilt grow fat.

Every tear from every eye
Becomes a babe in eternity;

The bleat, the bark, bellow, and roar,
Are waves that beat on heaven's shore.

— From "Auguries of Innocence" by William Blake

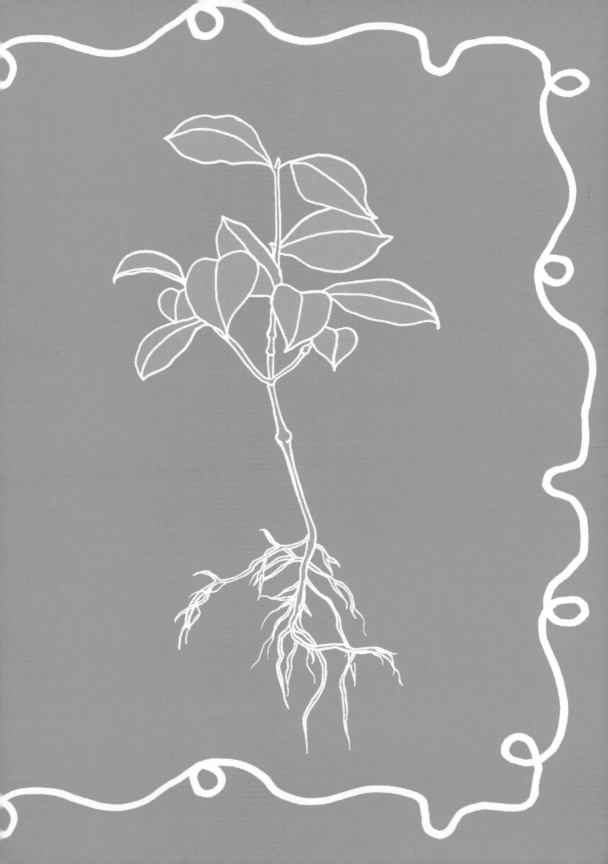

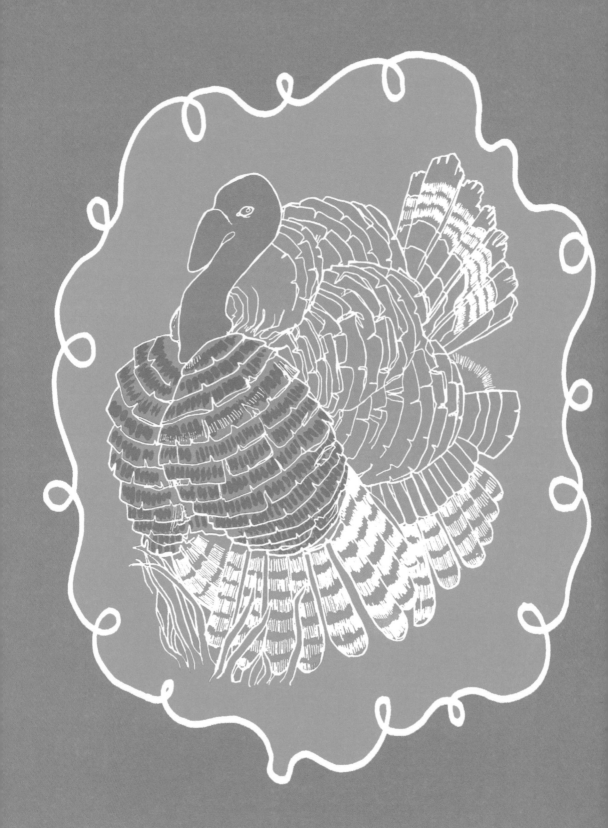

Notes

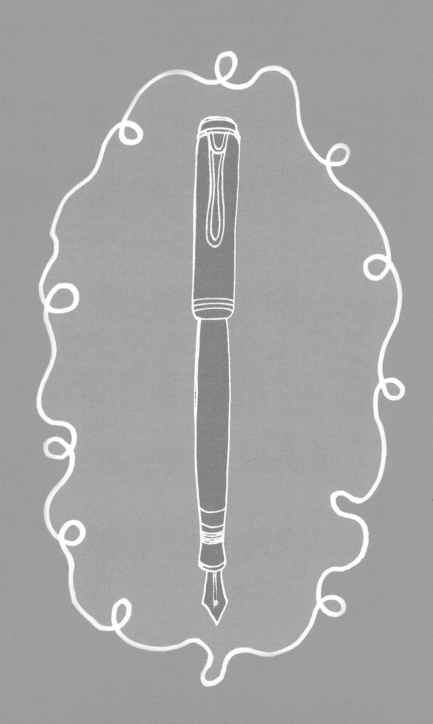

FINDING TIME FOR SILENCE

Consciously choosing to be silent is at once powerful and calming. Try it for a day. You may find great clarity and stillness in silence. Silence can also make you a better observer of the world around you. And when you break your silence, you may find that you're more thoughtful in the words you choose and the things you say. In the hours and days following your period of silence, did you see the world differently? Could you respond to others with more compassion?

NUTRITIONAL YEAST

A nonlive, nonactive yeast fermented on molasses, nutritional yeast has a cheesy flavor without the fat and dietary cholesterol. Use when making sauces and gravies; sprinkle it on popcorn, pasta or baked potatoes; or add it to a tofu scramble. A hint: Cats and dogs seem to love it as much as humans!

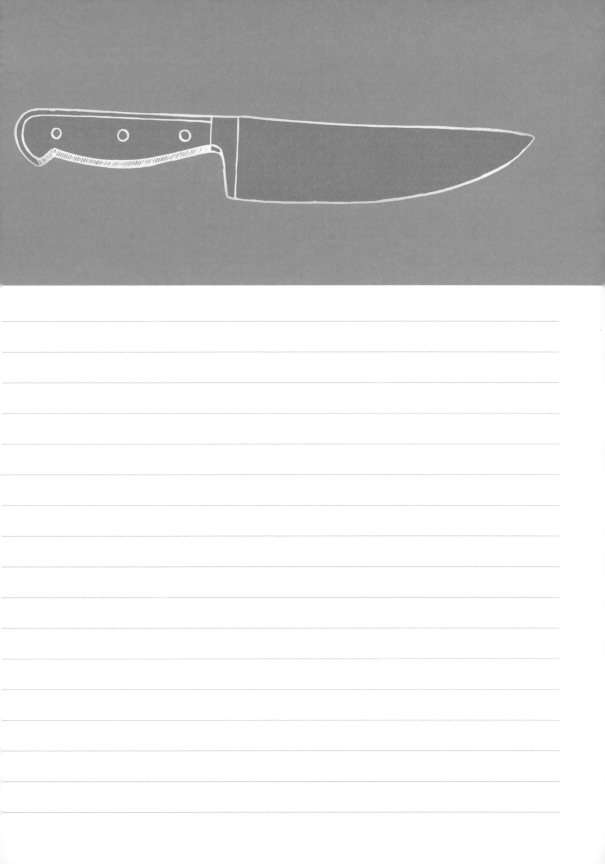

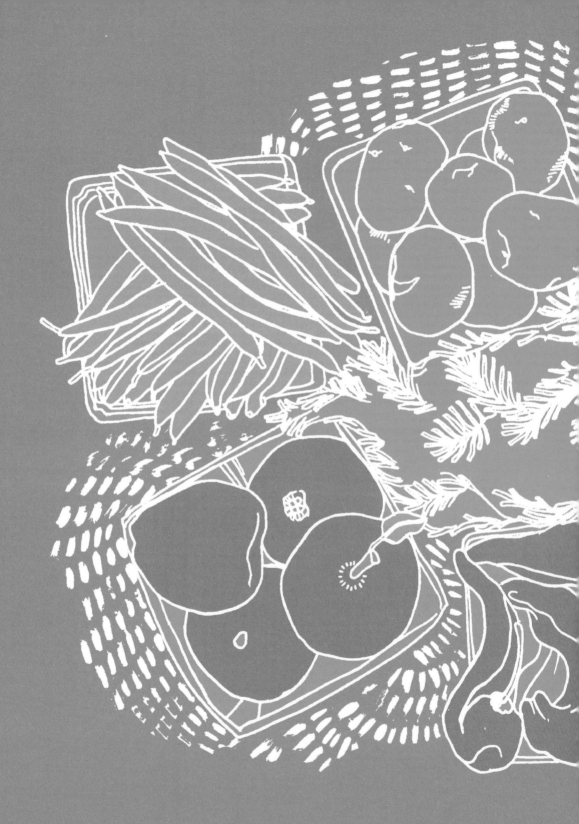

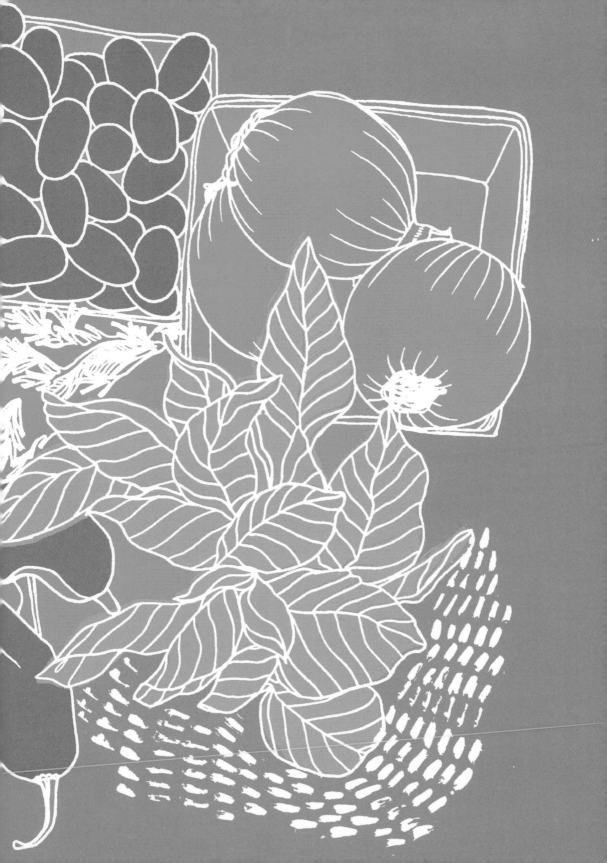

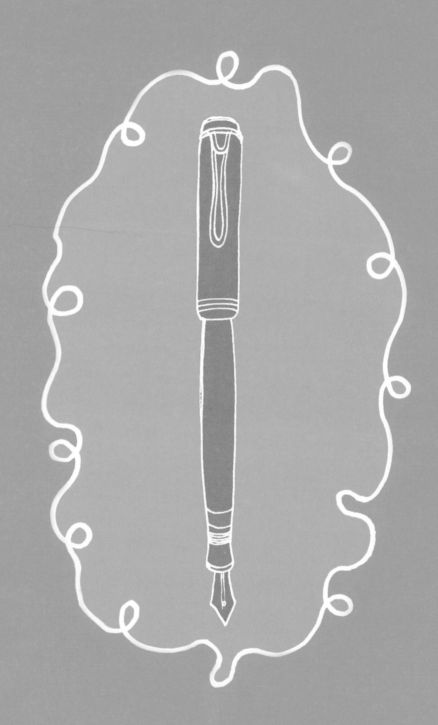

REMEMBERING YOUR STORY

When you are acutely aware of the vast consumption of animal products, it is easy to become frustrated by those participating in it. You may want to make others see what you see. But we can't force awareness. Remember that you, too, were once unaware. When someone saysa, "I just love meat too much to give it up," you might say, "I thought the same thing." How does the conversation change when you find common ground?

ON YOUR TABLE
QUINOA

Quinoa (pronounced KEEN-wa) is a staple in South America, where it has been grown in the Andes Mountains for more than 6,000 years. Be sure to rinse it before cooking to remove the bitter-tasting saponin. In your kitchen, this beautiful little seed can be enjoyed in many ways:

→ Cooked in vegetable broth and served with just a little salt and fresh herbs.
→ Mixed with corn kernels and steamed kale
→ In place of bulgur for a gluten-free version of tabbouleh
→ As a breakfast porridge, cooked as you would oatmeal, with almond milk and your favorite toppings

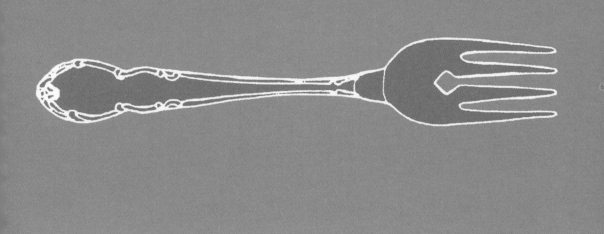
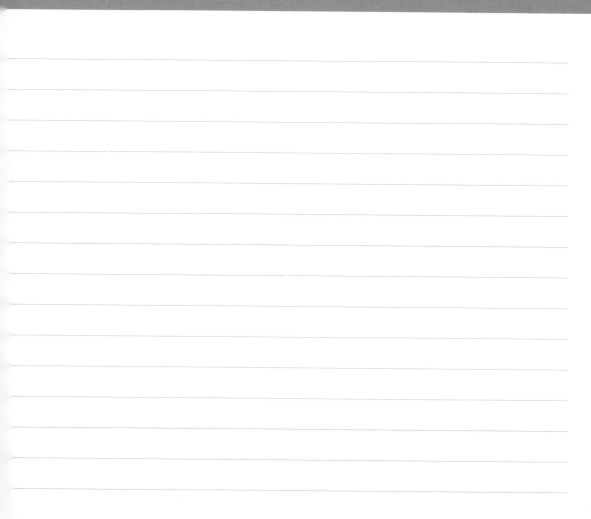

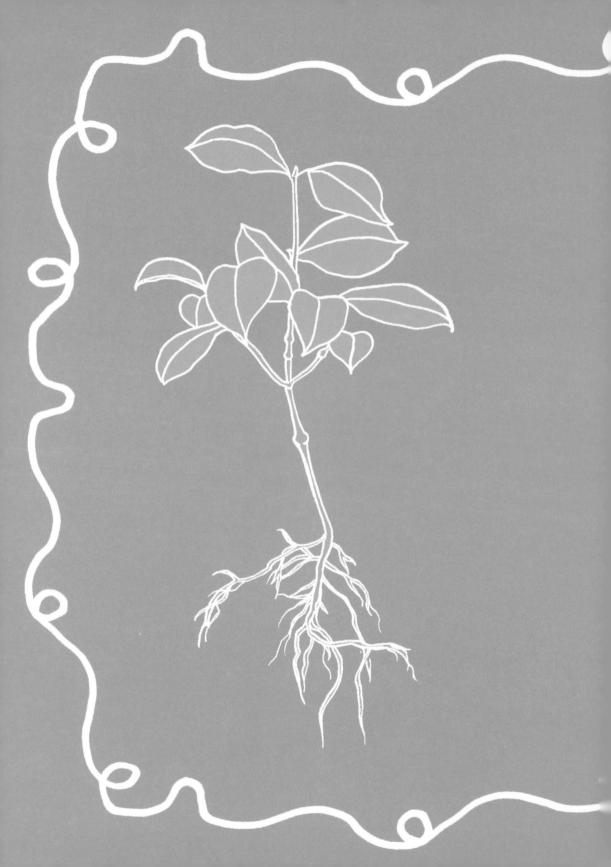

"My food is not that of man," says the creature. *"I do not destroy the lamb and kid to glut my appetite. Acorns and berries afford me sufficient nourishment. My companions will be of the same nature as myself and will be content with the same fare. We shall make our bed of dried leaves; the sun will shine on us as on man, and will ripen our food. The picture I present to you is peaceful and human, and you must feel that you could deny it only in the wantonness of power and cruelty."*

— From *Frankenstein* by *Mary Shelley*

Notes

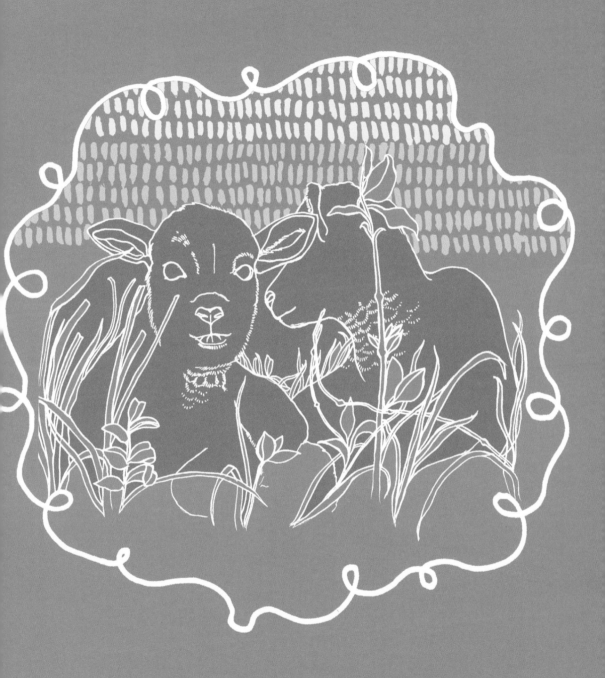

CONNECTING WITH LIKE-MINDED PEOPLE

Having a circle of like-minded people in your community—people you can dine with, who speak your language, who support your compassion for animals—is important. What do you do to connect with like-minded people?

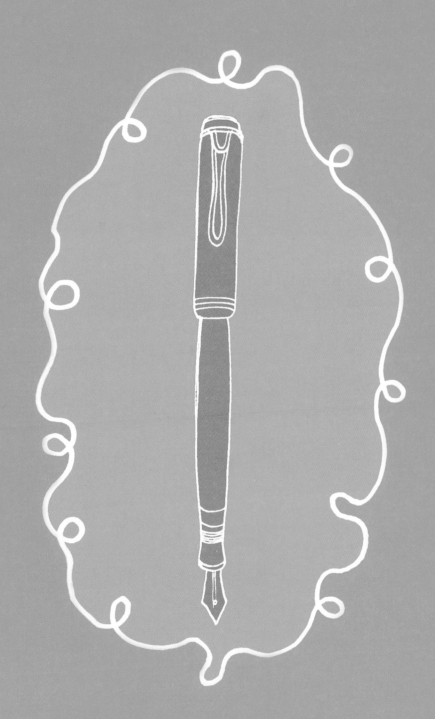

TEMPEH

Less familiar than its more popular soybean-based cousin, tofu, tempeh is made with whole soybeans fermented with grain. The process makes tempeh easier to digest, higher and protein, and higher in fiber than tofu. It also gives tempeh its nutty, earthy, slightly sweet flavor and firm, chewy texture. Steam tempeh before using it in a vegetable stir-fry, Mexican-style taco, or a pasta sauce.

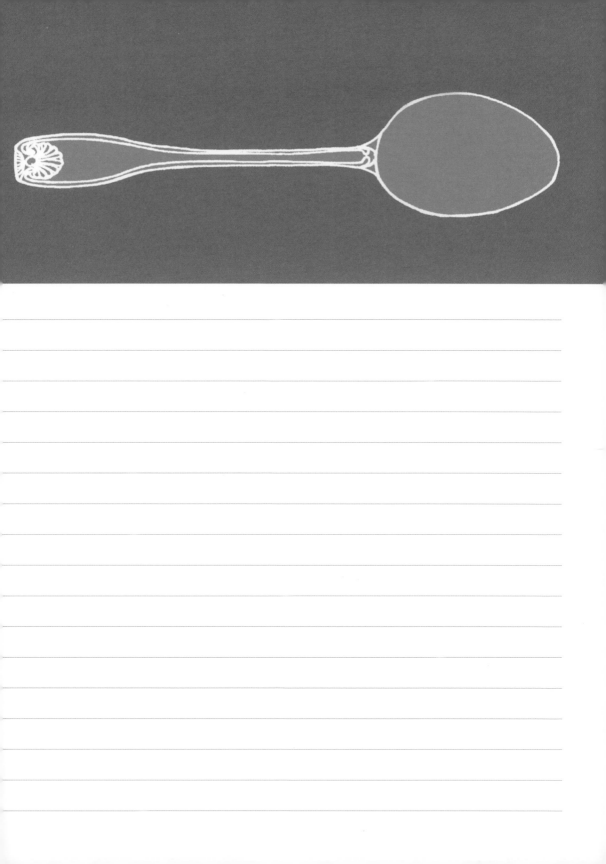

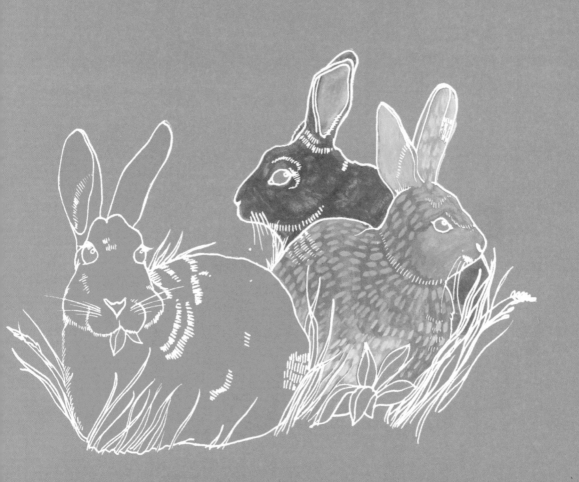

Notes

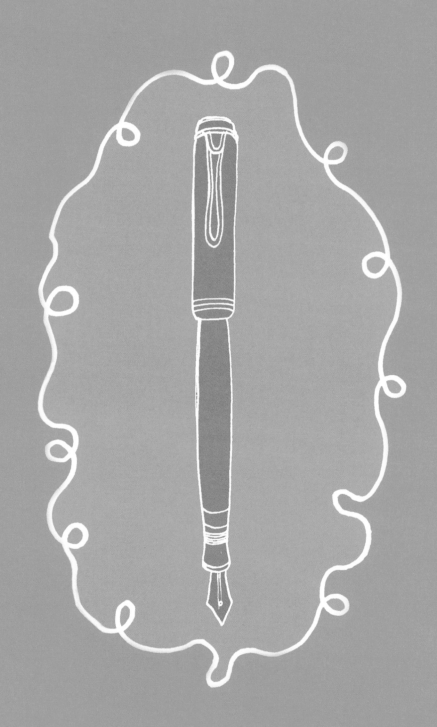

EXPRESSING GRATITUDE

Being grateful is really just about being aware of what is already in front of us—and taking a moment to acknowledge it. Making a gratitude list each day is a good way to practice being grateful. What are you grateful for right now?

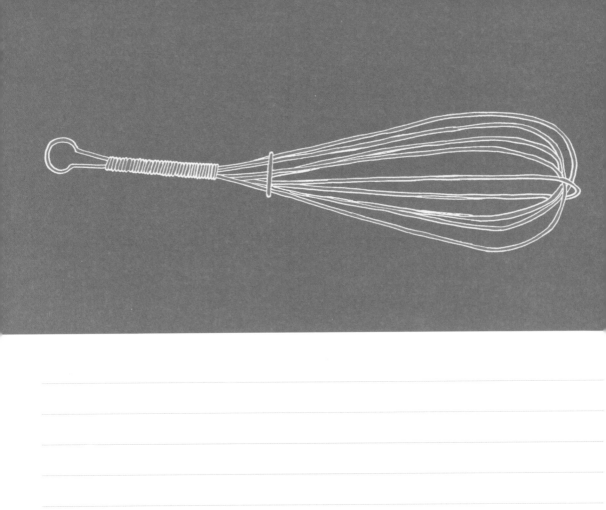
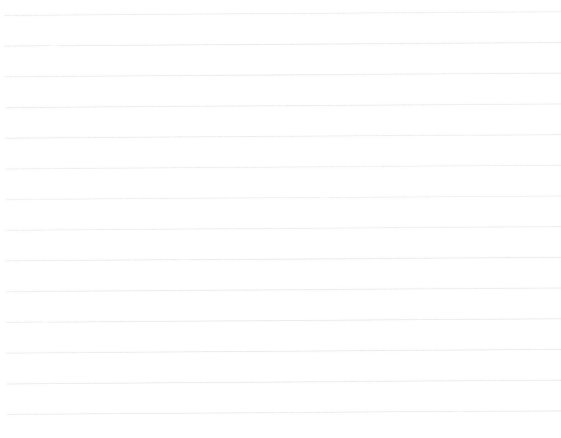

ON YOUR TABLE
DATES

Dates are nature's candy. The most common varieties are larger Medjool dates and smaller Deglet Noor dates. When using either variety, pit them before eating them as a low-calorie snack or adding them to fruit smoothies. Date sugar, made from ground, dehydrated dates, can be used to replace cane or beet sugar in many baking recipes.

Yes—thou mayst eat they bread, and lick the hand

That feeds thee; thou mayst frolic on the floor

At evening, and at night retire secure

To they straw couch, and slumber unalarm'd;

For I have gain'd they confidence, have pledged

All that is human in me, to protect

Thine unsuspecting gratitude and love.

If I survive thee, I will dig they grave;

And, when I place thee in it, sighing say,

I knew at least one hare that had a friend.

— From "My Pet Hare" by William Cowper

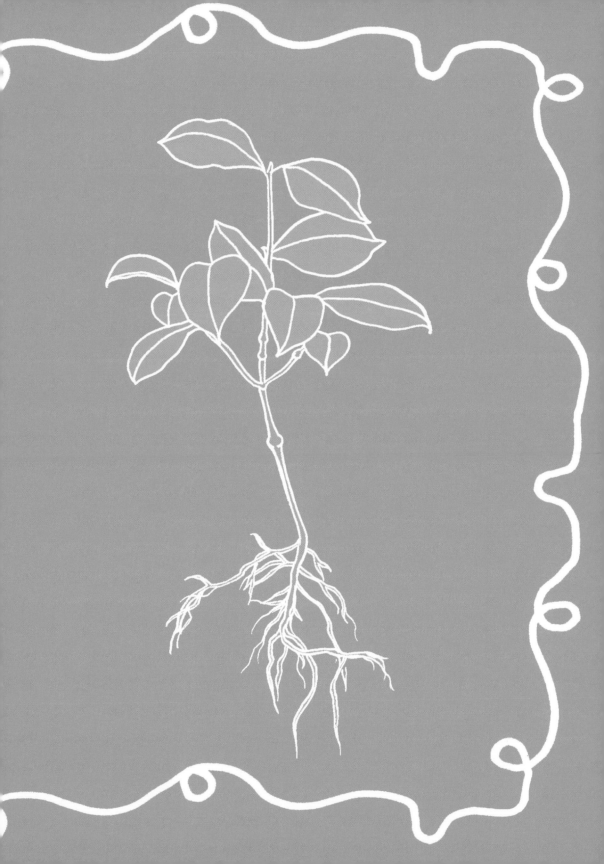

Notes

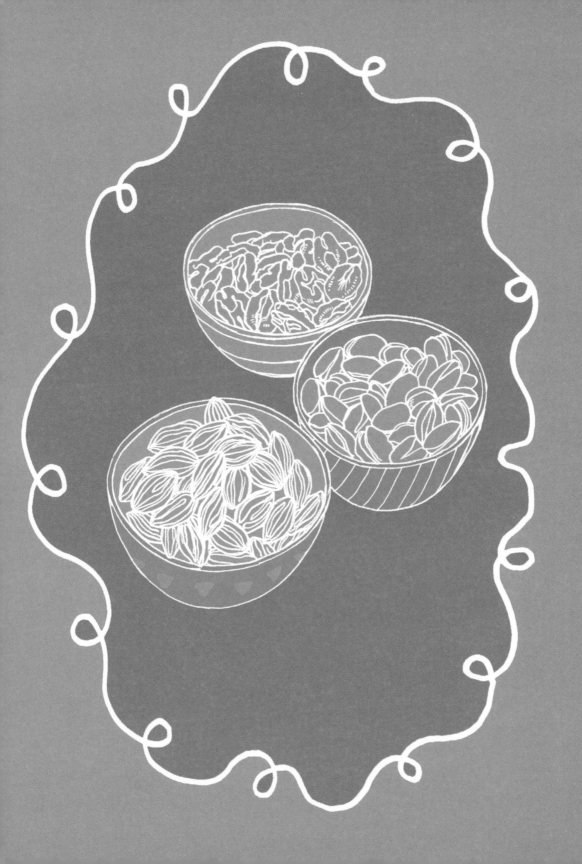

LISTENING

Being a good communicator doesn't just mean that you speak well; it also means that you listen well. Try to make listening an active—rather than passive—activity. Practice listening without thinking about what you want to say next. In listening attentively, can you see how relationships with those around you deepen?

DANDELION GREENS

In the Northern hemisphere, dandelions are considered a weed, but the plant's spicy leaves are delicious. Next time you see a dandelion, think dinner:

Dandelion greens are wonderful eaten raw as part of a salad.

Lightly boiled and sprinkled with salt and cider vinegar, they make an easy side dish.

They can be a spicier substitute for spinach, Swiss chard or kale in almost any dish.

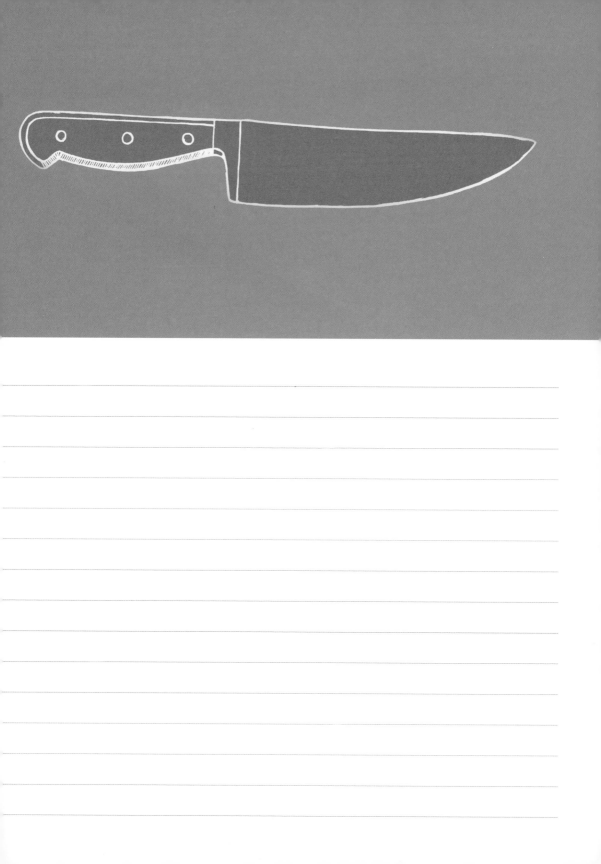

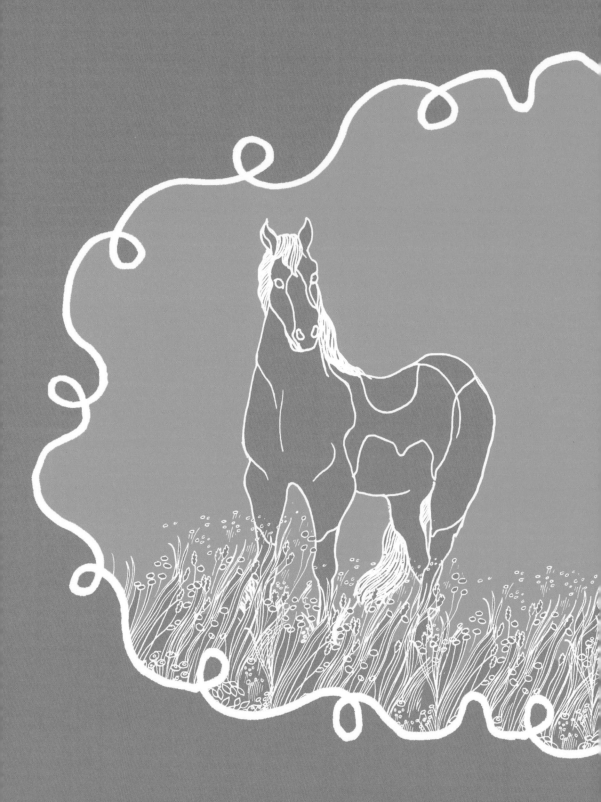

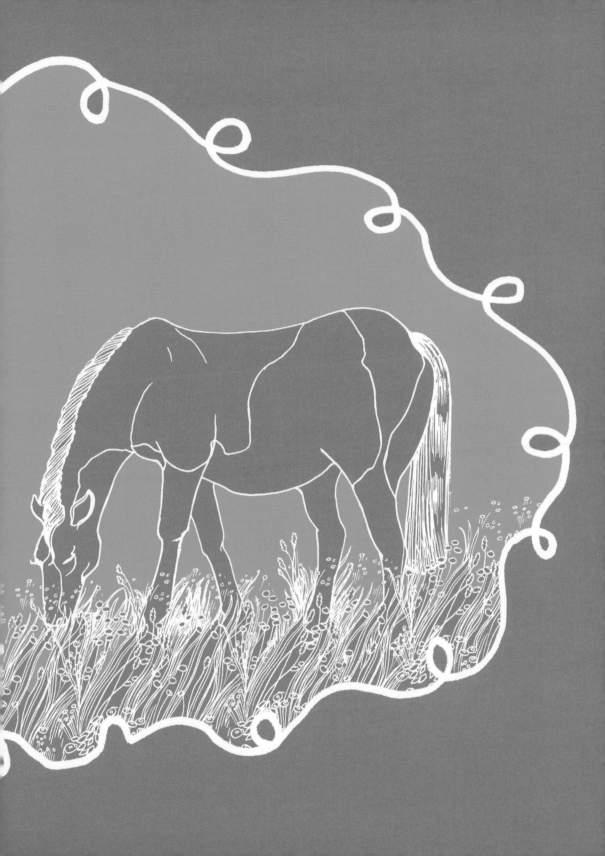

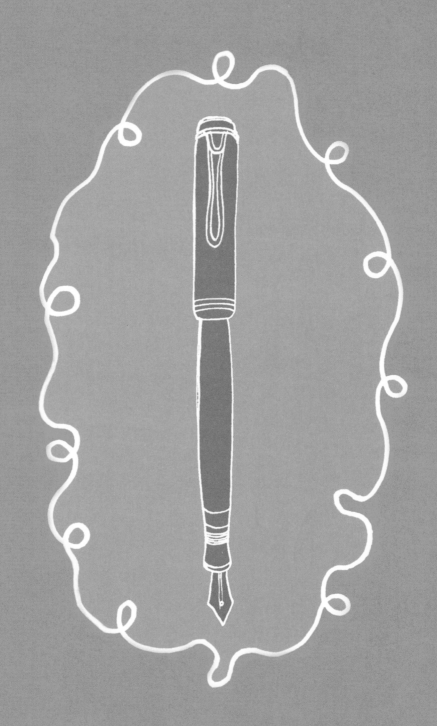

SPENDING TIME WITH ANIMALS

Research has found that interacting with animals may have physical and psychological benefits. If you don't live with an animal, you can visit a local animal sanctuary or volunteer at a rescue organization. Think about how you feel after you spend time with animals. Are you more relaxed? Happier?

ON YOUR TABLE
BARLEY

The oldest of all the grains, barley has a nutty flavor and a chewy texture. In the store you'll find three varieties: Scotch barley, with the bran intact; pot barley with part of the bran removed; and pearled barley with the hull and bran removed. Scotch is the most nutritious, but even pearled barley packs lots of iron and fiber. Add barley to soups, serve it alongside a stir-fry, or make a cold barley salad.

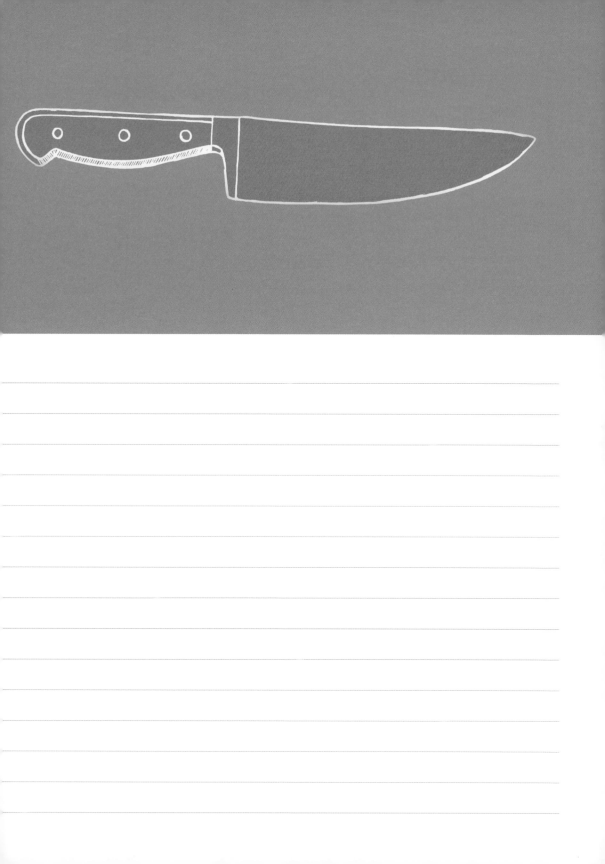

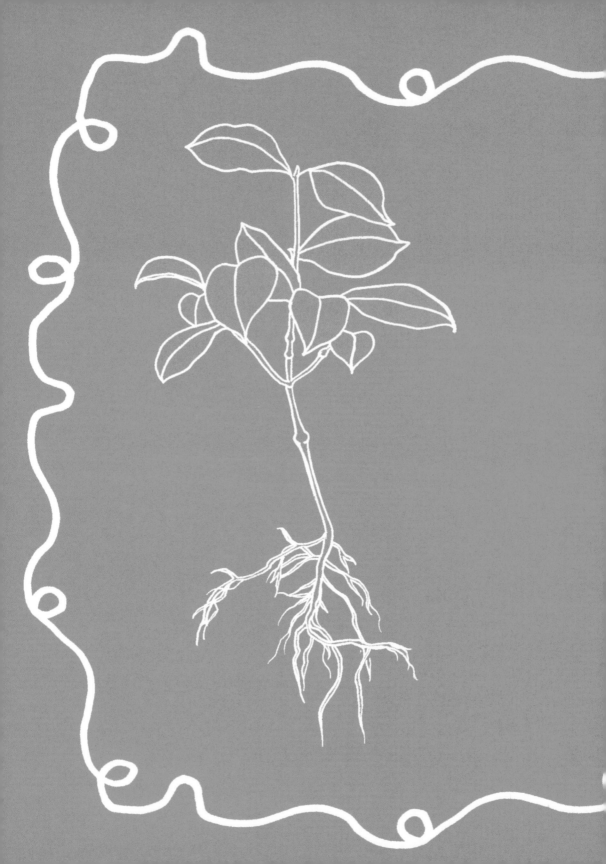

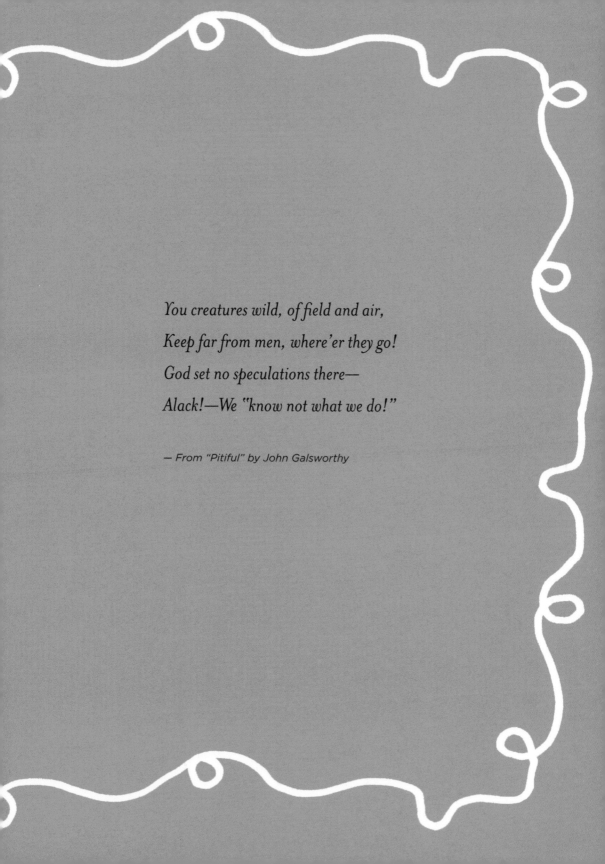

You creatures wild, of field and air,
Keep far from men, where'er they go!
God set no speculations there—
Alack!—We "know not what we do!"

— From "Pitiful" by John Galsworthy

Notes

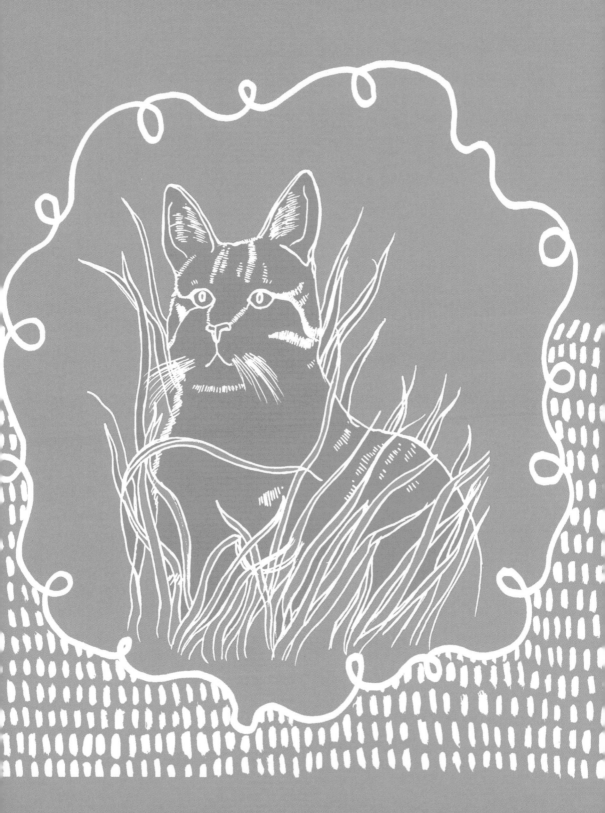

SETTING GOALS

There is something very powerful in declaring what you want—saying it out loud and writing it down. Creating goals and intentions is the first step to achieving them. What do you want?

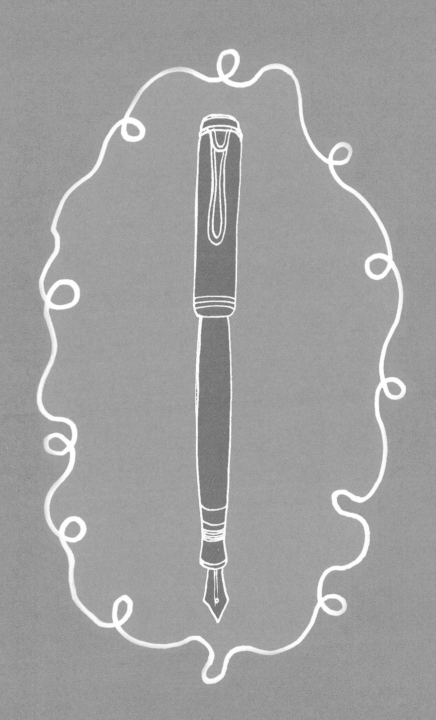

VINEGARS

Having a variety of vinegars in your cupboard means instant flavor.
Try a few of these delicious, versatile vinegars:

→ **APPLE CIDER VINEGAR:** a staple for quick dressings for green or
pasta salads. Look for raw apple cider vinegar for more flavor and
nutritional benefits

→ **BALSAMIC VINEGAR:** a sweet, complex vinegar. "Real," aged
balsamic is so syrupy you could eat it right off the spoon.

→ **WINE VINEGARS:** "everyday" vinegars. Pair red wine vinegar with
mushrooms and winter vegetables; white goes with lighter dishes.

→ **RICE VINEGAR:** mild, basic vinegar often used in Asian recipes.
Seasoned rice vinegar has a little sugar and goes well with greens.

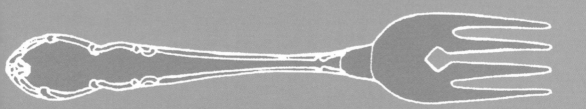

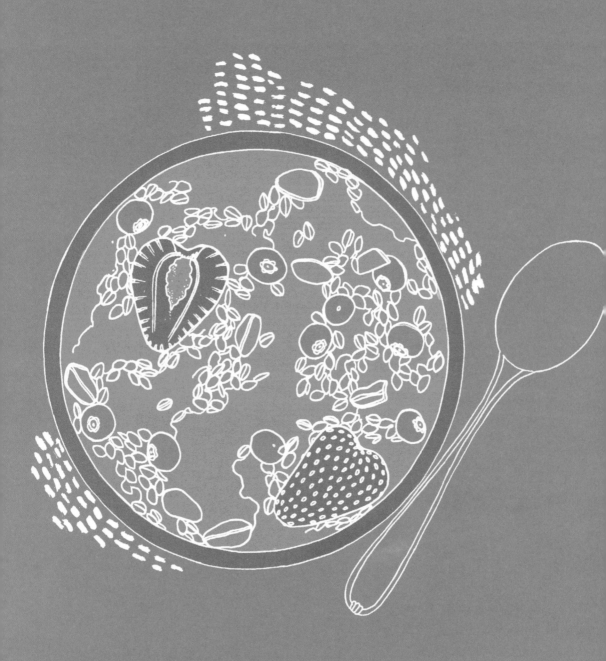

Notes

ASKING QUESTIONS

There are many myths and misconceptions about veganism, and vegans get a lot of questions from non-vegans. You won't know all the answers, but that's okay. Sometimes asking questions can be more powerful than offering answers. When someone says, "I could never be vegan," you might ask, "Why do you think it would be difficult for you?" What questions do you want to ask?

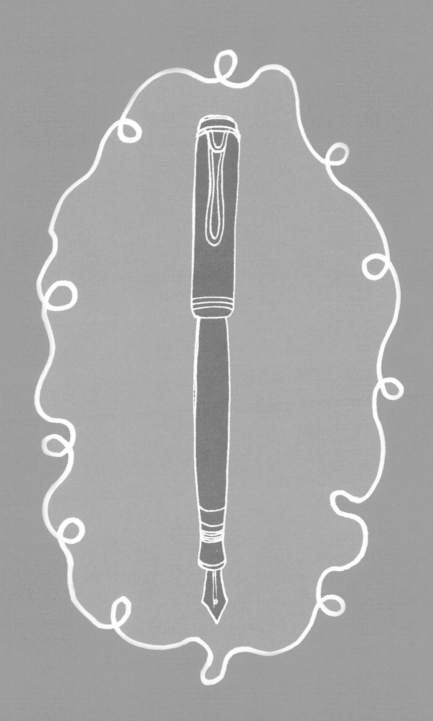

AGAR-AGAR

A gelatinous substance derived from red algae, agar-agar is often called "vegetarian gelatin." It's common in Japanese desserts, but it is also a useful substitute to animal-based gelatin, which is made from the boiled remains of bones, skin, and connective tissues of slaughterhouse victims. Hint: Some recipes use agar-agar as a thickener, but arrowroot, kudzu root, and cornstarch work just as well.

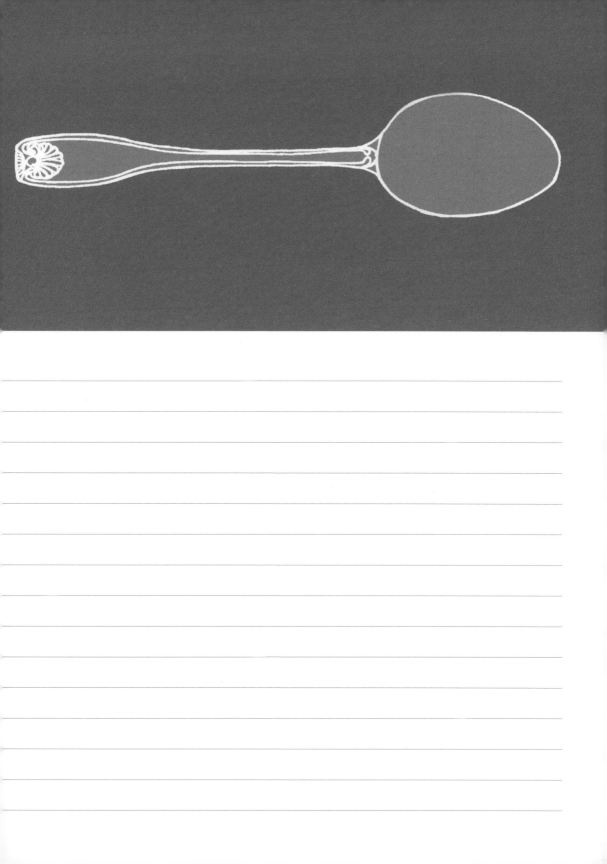

In England once there lived a big
And wonderfully clever pig.
To everybody it was plain
That Piggy had a massive brain.
He worked out sums inside his head,
There was no book he hadn't read.
He knew what made an airplane fly,
He knew how engines worked and why.
He knew all this, but in the end
One question drove him round the bend:
He simply couldn't puzzle out

What LIFE was really all about.
What was the reason for his birth?
Why was he placed upon this earth?
His giant brain went round and round.
Alas, no answer could be found.
Till suddenly one wondrous night.
All in a flash he saw the light.
He jumped up like a ballet dancer
And yelled, "By gum, I've got the answer!
They want my bacon slice by slice
To sell at a tremendous price!"

— From "Pig" by Roald Dahl

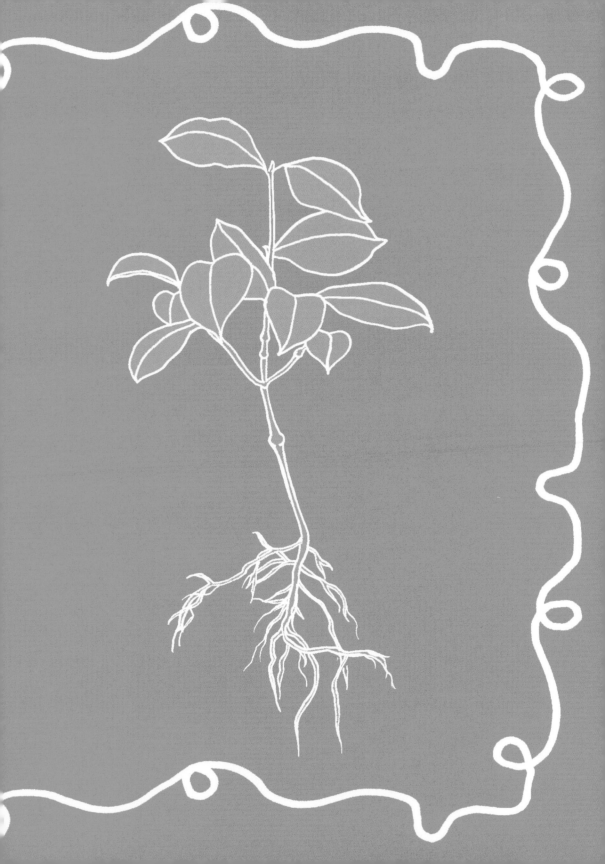

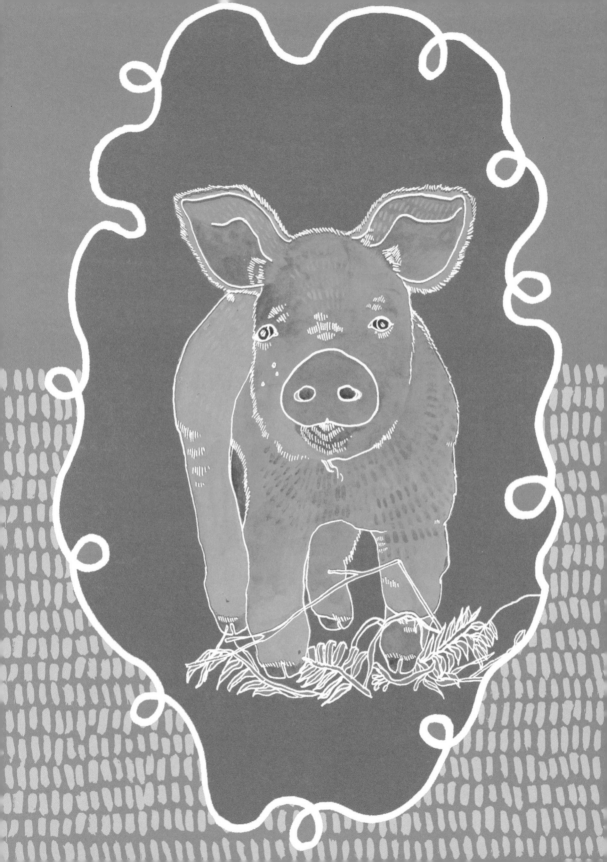

Notes

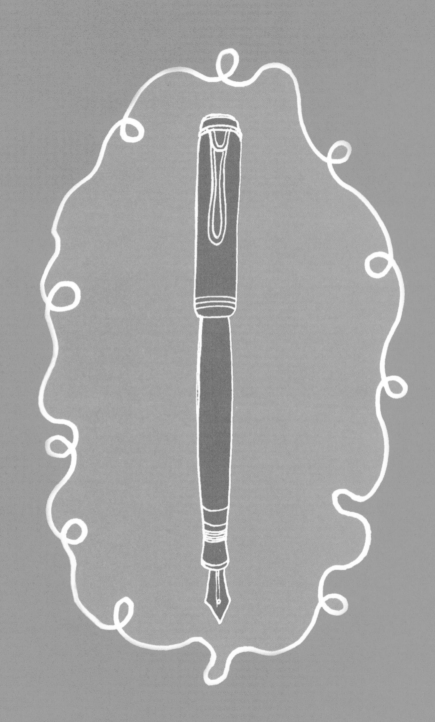

EATING MORE WHOLE FOODS

The most healthful diet you can eat is one based on whole foods—foods that are as close to their natural state as possible. Although there is a spectrum of "processed foods," every time you choose something that is highly processed you are missing out on the benefits of a healthful whole food. What is in your kitchen? What changes do you want to make?

CACAO NIBS

Chocolate is vegan! It comes from the seeds of the cacao tree. And cocoa nibs—pieces of the cacao seeds—are as delicious as a snack as they are in your favorite baked goods. Raw, they taste like very dark chocolate. Roasted, they have a smoky flavor similar to roasted coffee beans.

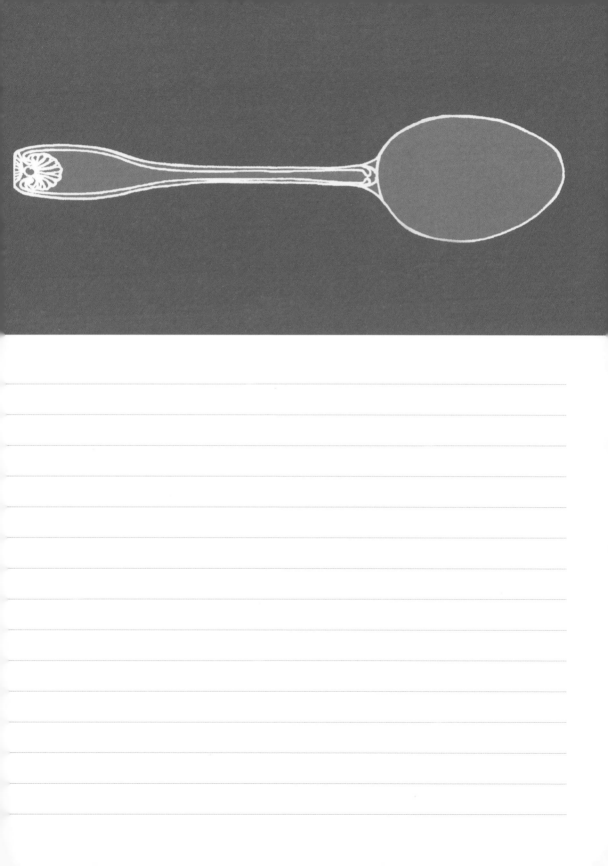

Notes

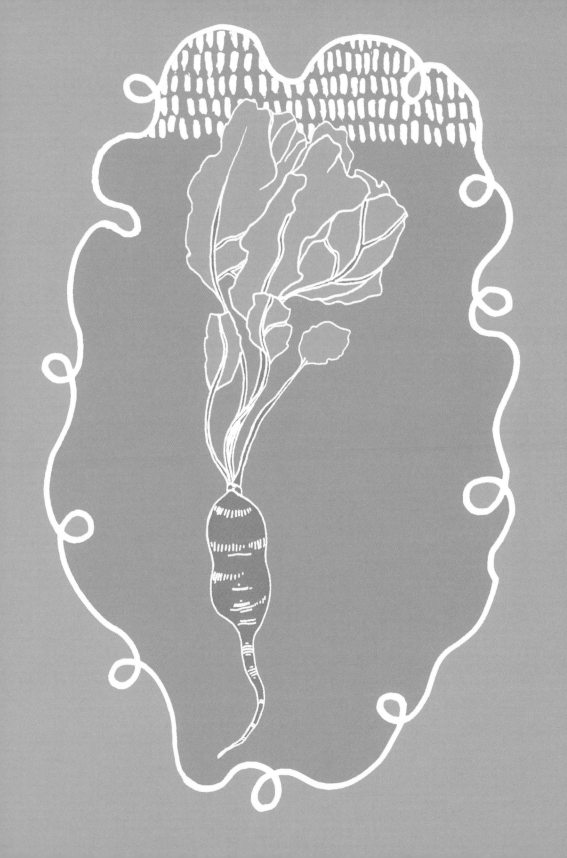

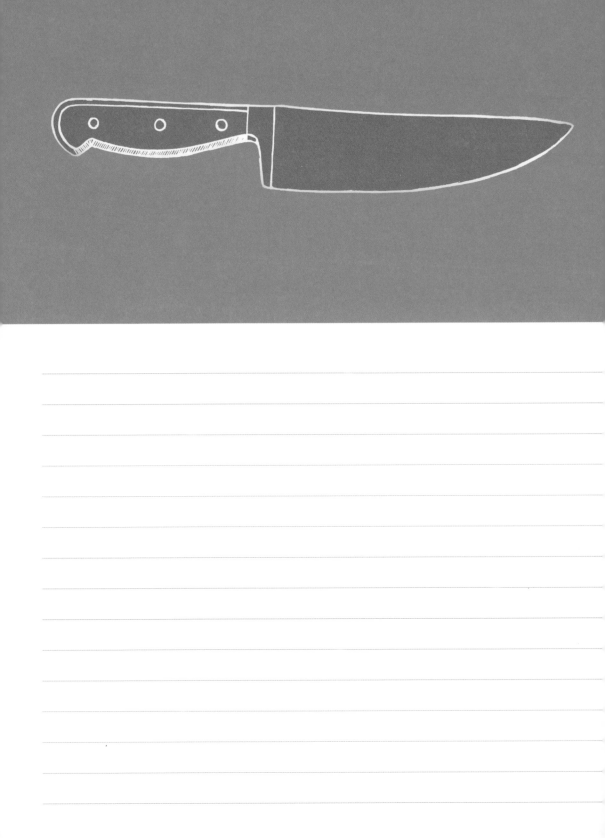

KNOWING YOUR LIMITATIONS

Bearing witness to violence against animals—via undercover investigations, documentaries, or in person—can be a difficult thing to experience, and yet it's what so many of us needed to become aware. How do you find balance between staying connected to the truth and healing from the trauma of witnessing atrocities against animals? How do you take care of yourself?

SEA VEGETABLES

"Sea vegetables" is the more accurate—and more appetizing—name for seaweed. Sea vegetables are popular in Japan. Seek out these impressively nutritious plants:

→ **SPIRULINA:** rich in minerals. It can be found as a food supplement in natural food stores and is often added to fruit smoothies for a green color and a nutrient boost.

→ **KOMBU:** the best-known species of kelp, used to make soup stock or added to cooking beans to increase digestibility.

→ **WAKAME:** calcium- and iron-rich species of kelp, is frequently found in soups and salads.

→ **NORI:** a general term of edible seaweed of the genus *Porphrya*. It's an integral part of sushi and it's also delicious in a salad.

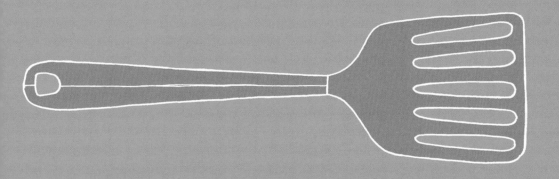

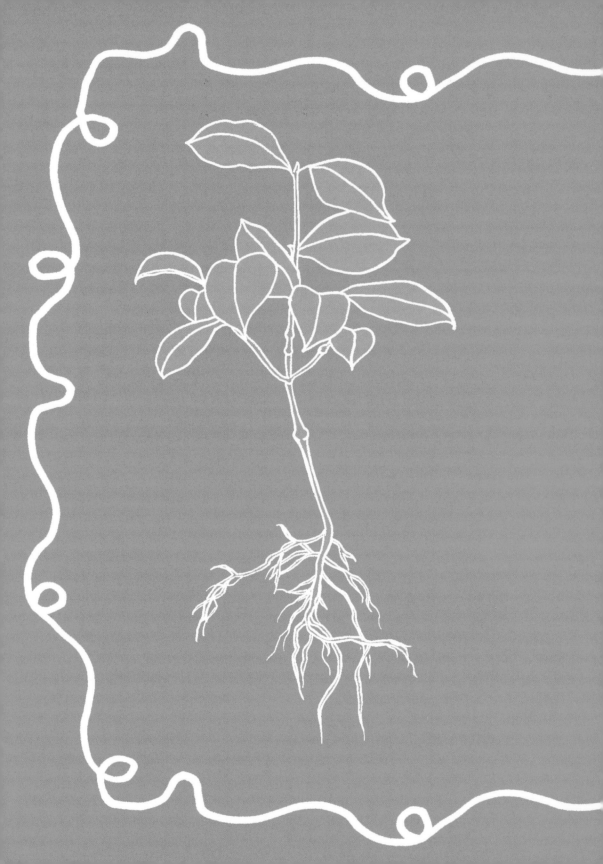

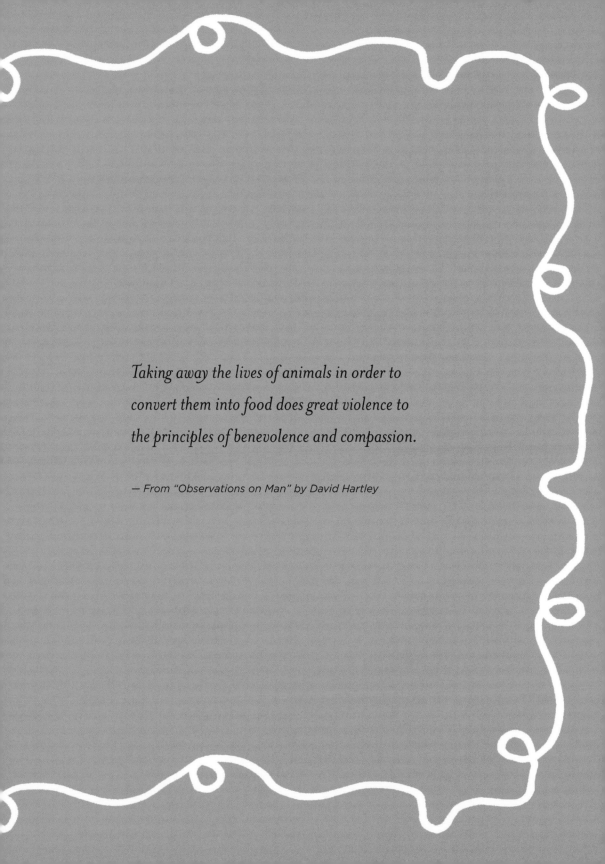

Taking away the lives of animals in order to convert them into food does great violence to the principles of benevolence and compassion.

— From "Observations on Man" by David Hartley

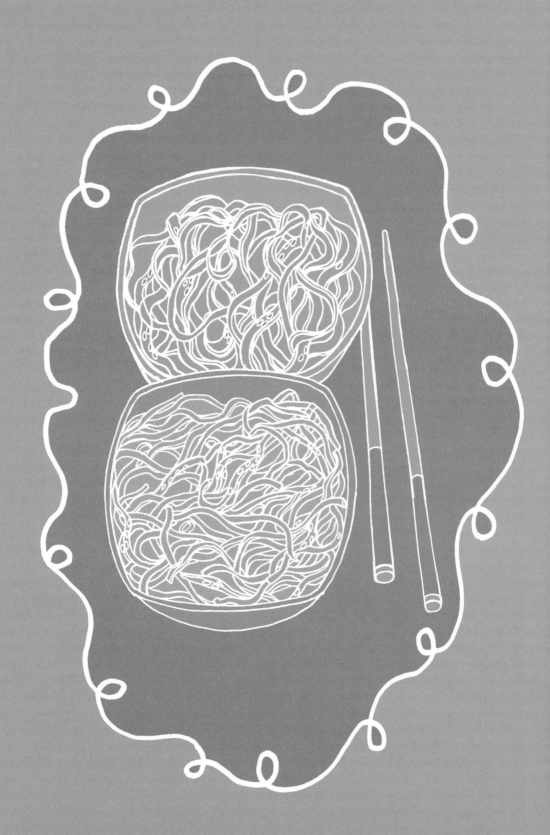

Notes

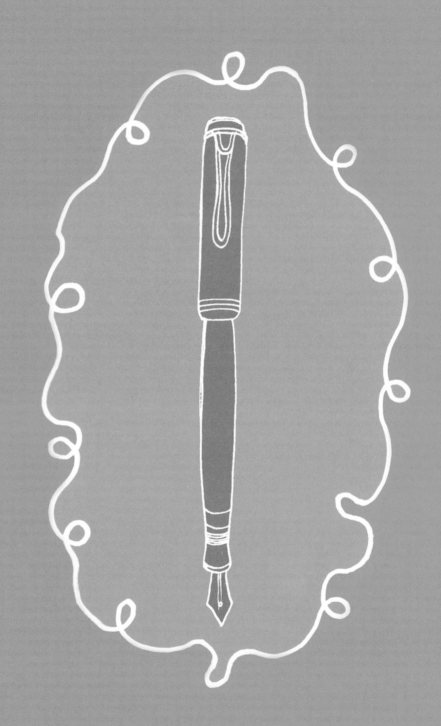

CONSIDERING YOUR WORDS

How often do you use or hear unappetizing words like "faux," "mock," "imitation," or "analogue" in relation to "vegan food"? Not only do these words make plant-based food seem inferior to animal-based products, but also they can turn people away from what is an abundant and delicious way to live. What positive words can you use and encourage when talking about this way of being in the world?

TAHINI

Whereas peanut butter is made from ground peanuts, tahini is made from ground sesame seeds. Common in traditional Middle Eastern cuisine (such as hummus), tahini can be used to make a simple sauce or salad dressing. It adds a creamy component to vegetable purees, and it thickens soups and stews. It's even great in desserts: Mix tahini and agave nectar, and dip bread into the sweet concoction.

Notes

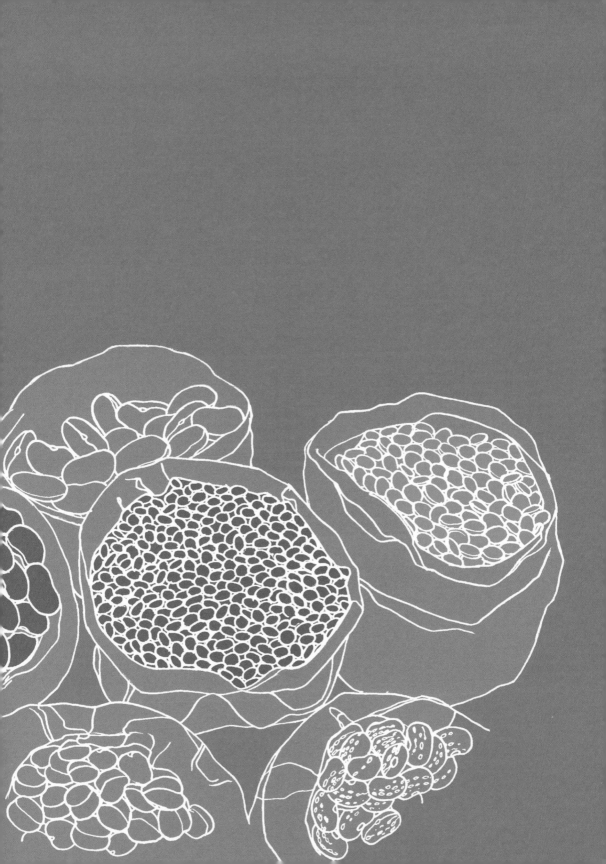

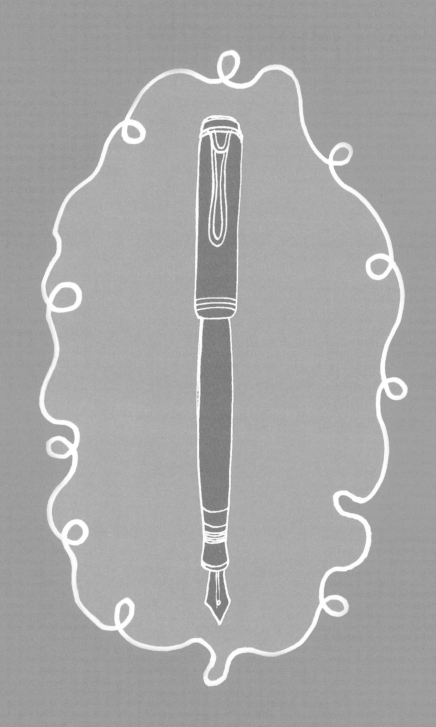

CREATING A SACRED SPACE

Everyone craves a place of retreat. Do you have a place where you can withdraw to rejuvenate and relax? Choose a comfortable, intimate place and make it your own by filling it with objects that hold special meaning for you. What feeling do you want to evoke in your special sanctuary? How do you want to feel?

COCONUTS

You need fat in your diet to absorb various fat-soluble nutrients. Coconuts can provide a source of that fat in a healthful diet. Experiment with coconut in many forms:

→ **COCONUT MILK:** sweet, thick milk used for rich dishes like Thai curries and desserts. It can be used in place of other milks in baking.

→ **COCONUT OIL AND BUTTER:** for use in sautéing vegetables or making baked goods.

→ **DRIED COCONUT:** available shredded or in flakes. It is great for baking or in fruit salad, oatmeal, and trail mix.

→ **COCONUT WATER:** the juice of a young coconut. It has no fat, but it makes a refreshing drink.

→ **COCONUT MEAT:** the flesh of a young coconut. Coconut meat is great for snacking.

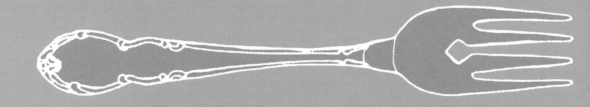

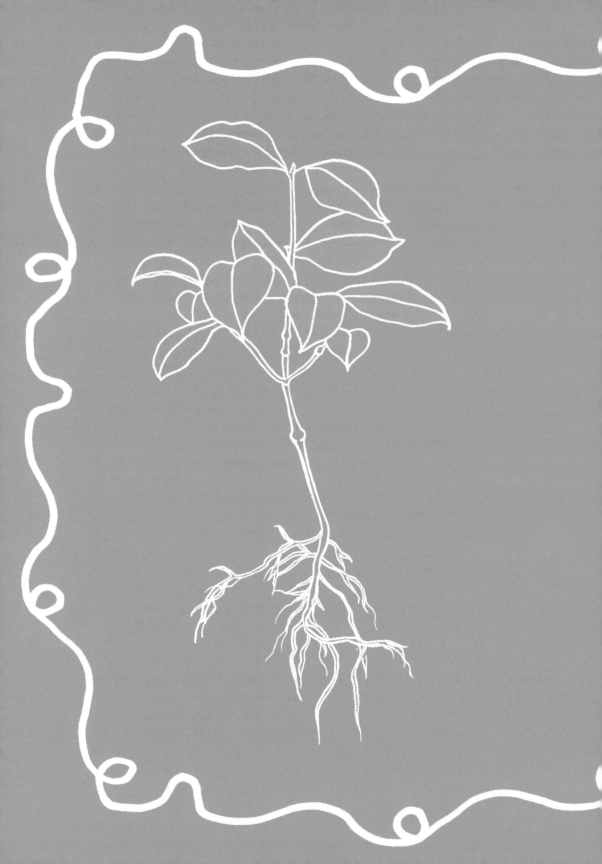

Take any bird, put it in a cage, and set your mind and heart all on fostering it tenderly with food and drink, with all dainty things you can imagine, and keep it as cleanly as you can; even if its cage may be ever so delightful with gold, this bird would still twenty thousand times rather go eat worms and other such wretched things from the cold and crude forest. For he will do his best at all times to escape from his cage, if he can; this bird always desires his liberty.

— From "The Canterbury Tales" by Geoffrey Chaucer

Notes

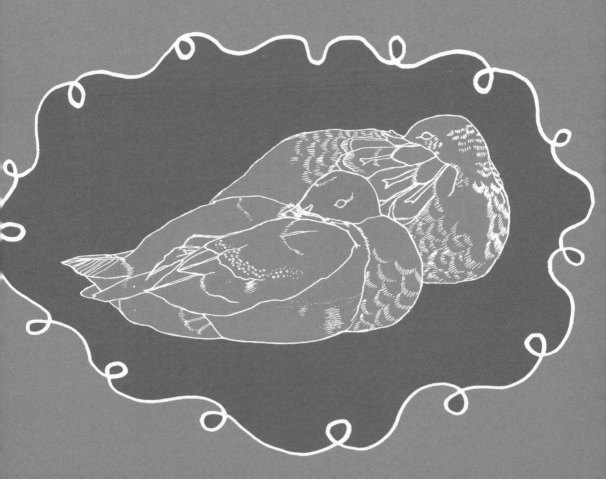

CRYING

Shedding a few tears can provide the relief and healing necessary to feel empowered, strong, and refreshed after witnessing images of animal abuse. How do you cope with sadness? Do you let yourself cry? Do you feel the need to apologize when you do? How can you own your tears?

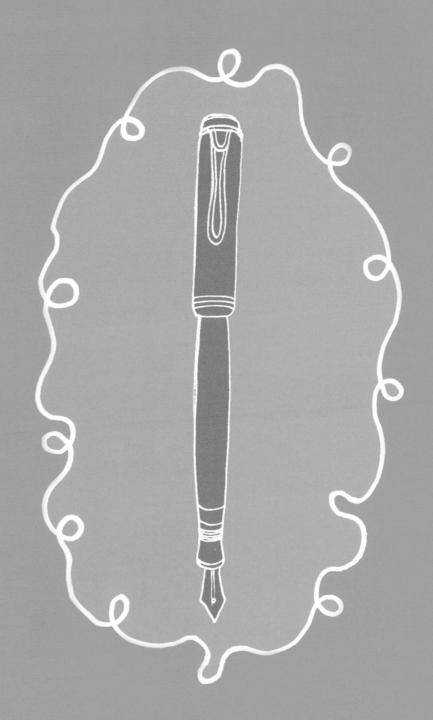

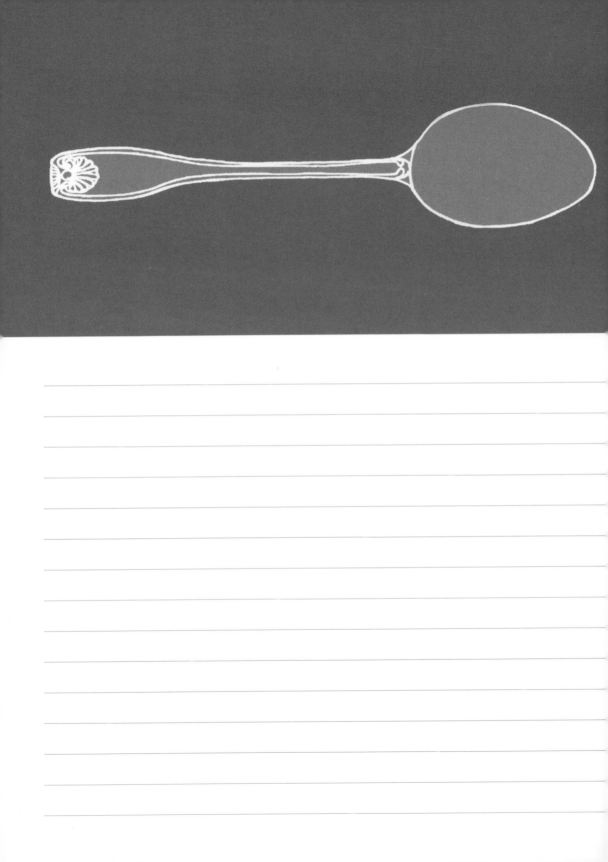

SEITAN

This wheat-based food has many names: wheat gluten, grain meat, wheat meat, gluten meat, "mock" meat, or seitan (pronounced SAY-tan.) A chewy, protein-rich food, seitan is usually marinated and then stir-fried, grilled, baked, barbecued, or fried. It's also the main ingredient in many commercial vegan meats. In what ways do you prepare this ancient grain meat?

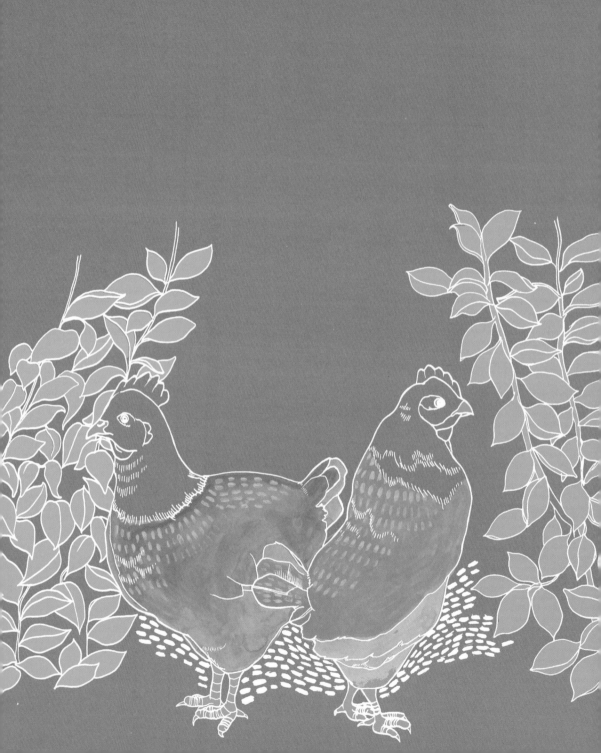

Notes

ADMITTING WHEN YOU DON'T KNOW

When someone asks you a question about veganism, animal rights, or nutrition that you don't know the answer to, how do you respond? Do you feel you have to be an expert in nutrition, philosophy, animal husbandry, history, ecology, and the culinary arts? Sometimes just saying, "I don't know" is a perfectly acceptable answer. How do you use humility in your advocacy?

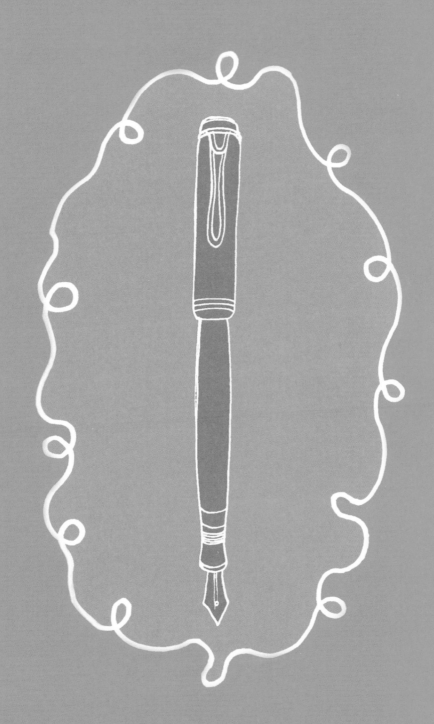

ON YOUR TABLE
MISO

A traditional Japanese food, miso is created by fermenting rice, barley, and/or soybeans with salt into a thick paste used in soups, dressings, soups, and spreads. It provides instant flavor and nutrition. Different lengths of fermentation create different flavors:

→ **WHITE MISO:** sweet; used in salad dressings, light sauces, and soups

→ **YELLOW MISO:** mild, earthy; used in sauces, marinades, dressings, and soups

→ **RED MISO:** dark, rich; used in hearty soups, glazes, and marinades.

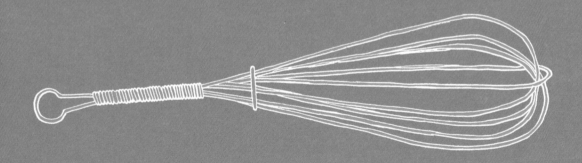

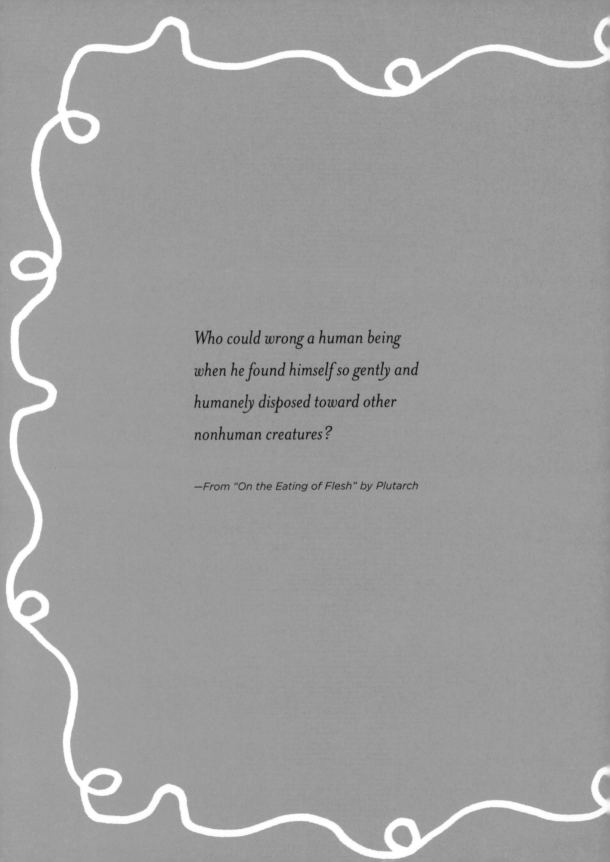

*Who could wrong a human being
when he found himself so gently and
humanely disposed toward other
nonhuman creatures?*

—From "On the Eating of Flesh" by Plutarch

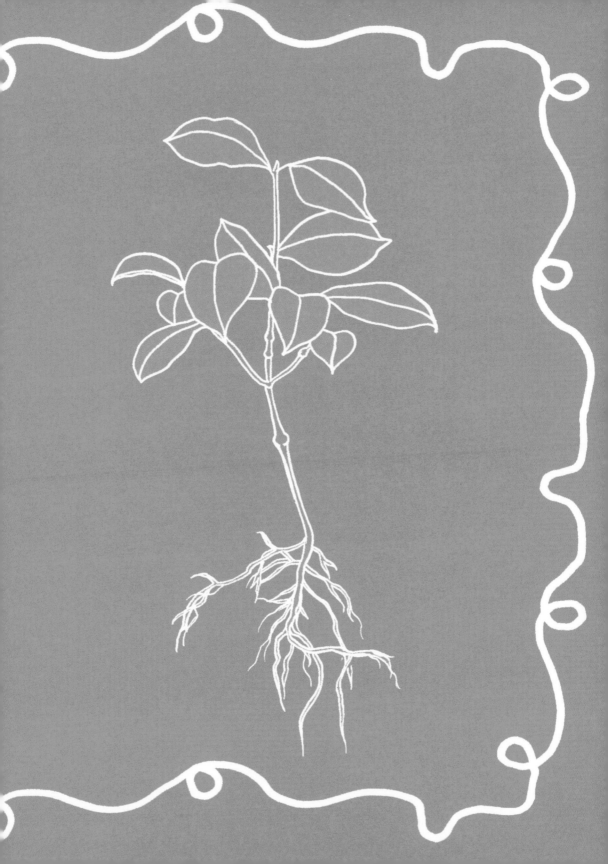

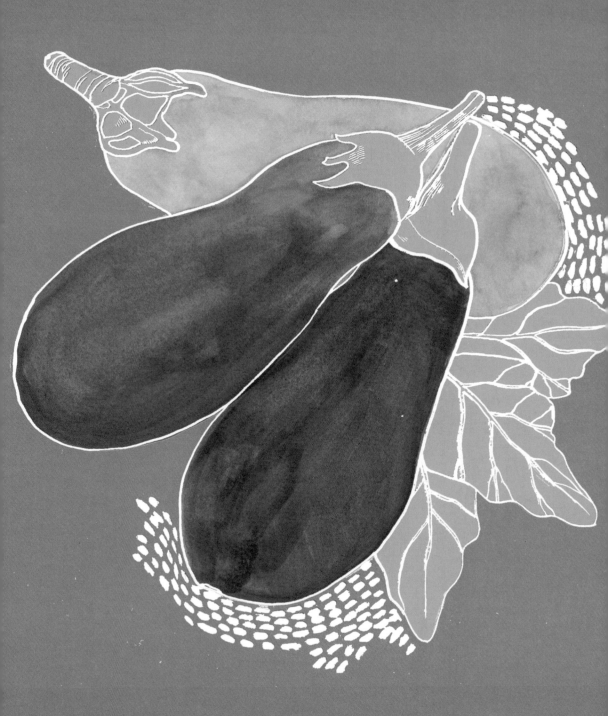

Notes

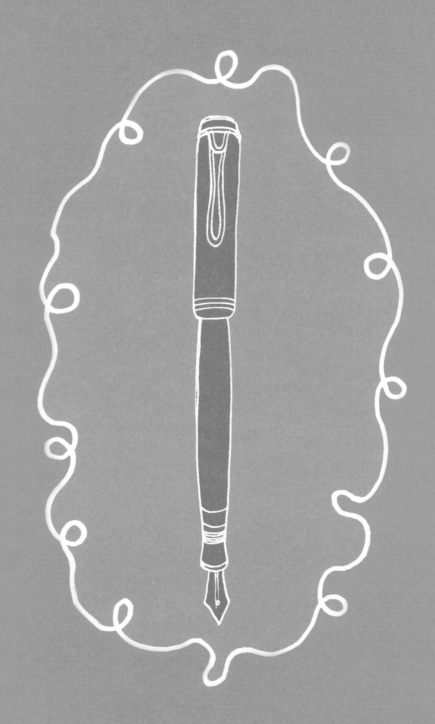

SPENDING TIME IN NATURE

Time spent outdoors can be incredibly restorative. It connects you with the more fundamental cycles of life and engages the senses. Have you been outside today? Take a walk or simply do outside whatever you usually do inside, whether it's eating, cooking, yoga, meditation, reading, or working.

SEEDS

An excellent source of fiber, protein, selenium, and vitamin E, seeds can be a regular part of a healthful diet. It's true they are high in fat, but most of it is monounsaturated fat, and that's a good thing. Flaxseeds, hemp seeds, pumpkin seeds, sesame seeds, sunflower seeds, and chia seeds are great pantry additions.

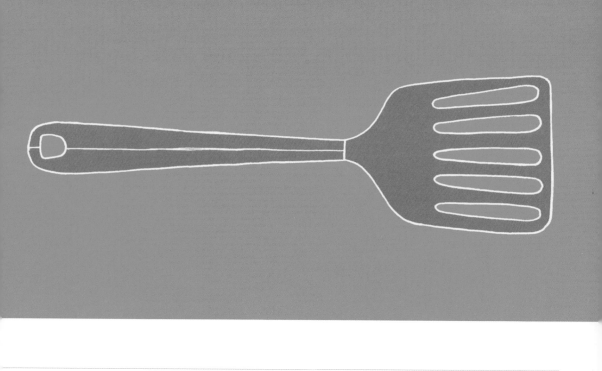

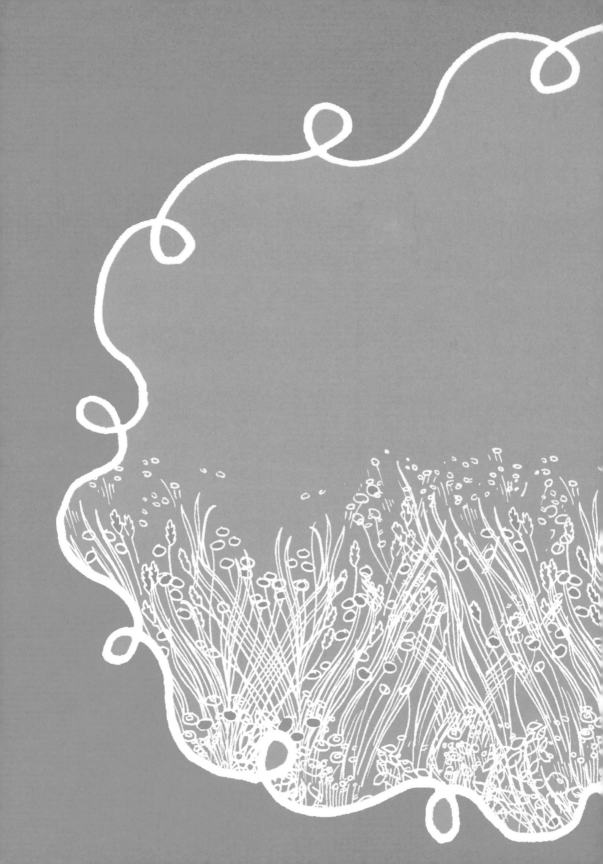

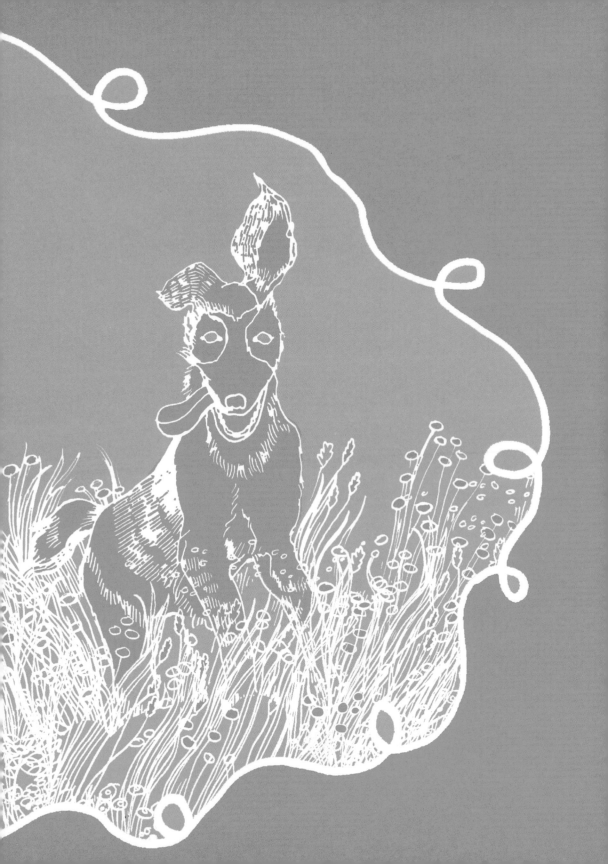

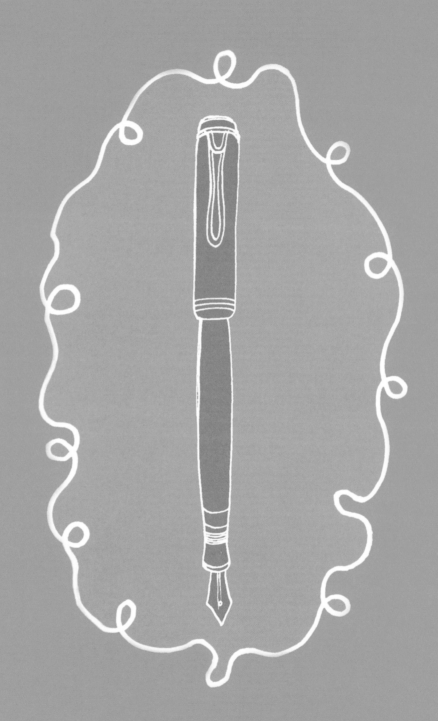

LAUGHING

When you're aware of the suffering so many billions of animals endure every day, it's easy to get swallowed up by the sorrow it induces. Feeling that pain is essential, but so is laughing. It lowers the blood pressure, relaxes the body, boosts the immune system, and releases endorphins. Do you feel guilty when you laugh knowing animals are suffering? Can you give yourself permission to laugh and still be an effective advocate?

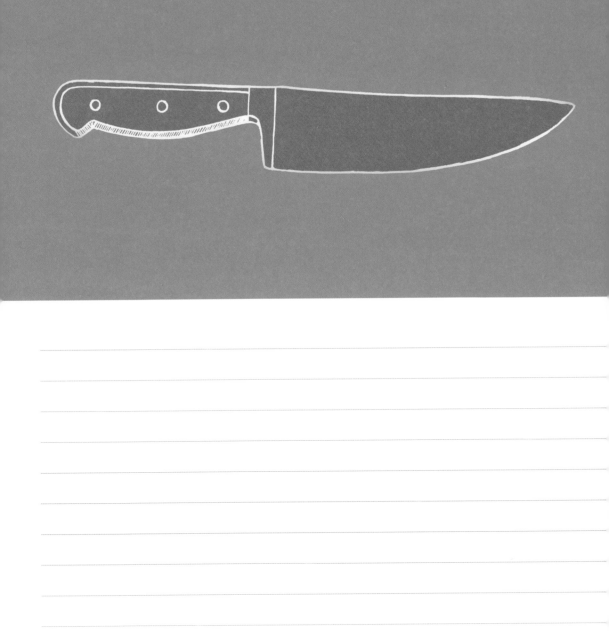

ON YOUR TABLE
WALNUTS

Walnuts are a wonderful source of omega-3 fatty acids and protein.
They are also incredibly versatile. Try them in oatmeal, on a salad, in
granola or trail mix, sautéed with vegetables, coarsely chopped on top
of soup or pasta, or mixed with chopped fruit and nondairy yogurt. Or
just eat them as a snack.

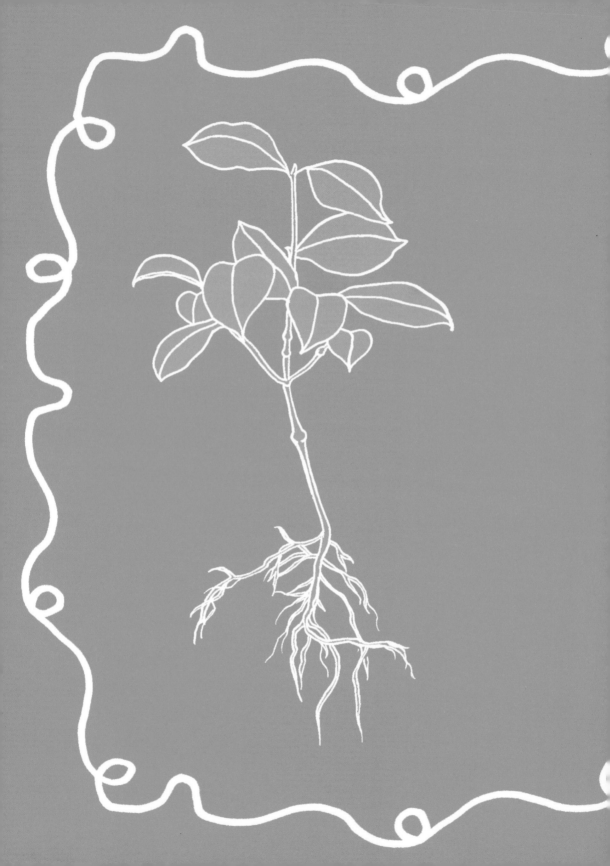

I think I could turn and live with animals, they are so placid and self-contain'd,
I stand and look at them long and long.

They do not sweat and whine about their condition,
They do not lie awake in the dark and weep for their sins,
They do not make me sick discussing their duty to God,
Not one is dissatisfied, not one is demented with the mania of owning things,
Not one kneels to another, nor to his kind that lived thousands of years ago,
Not one is respectable or unhappy over the whole earth.

— From "Leaves of Grass" by Walt Whitman

Notes

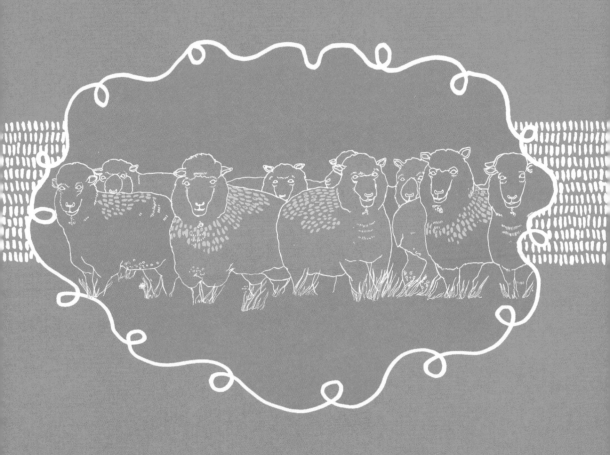

ASKING FOR WHAT YOU WANT

How do you respond when someone serves you something non-vegan in his or her home? Some people feel it is rude to decline something that is offered, but why should someone else's comfort level be more important than our own principles—and our own desire for a satisfying dinner? A simple conversation before dinner can usually prevent an awkward moment. Have you given yourself permission to ask for what you want without being apologetic or self-effacing? What are some ways you practice this?

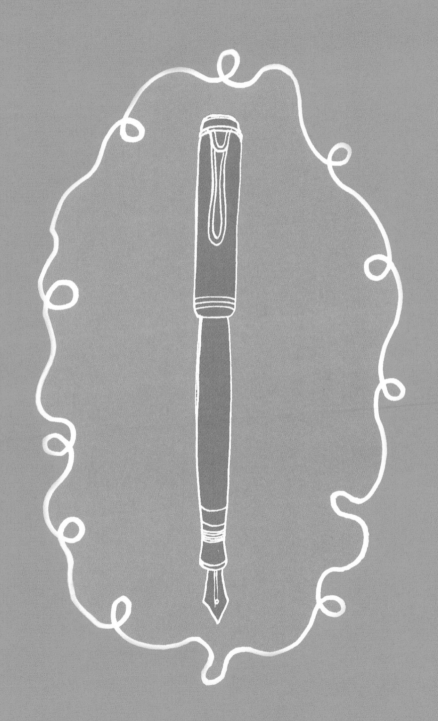

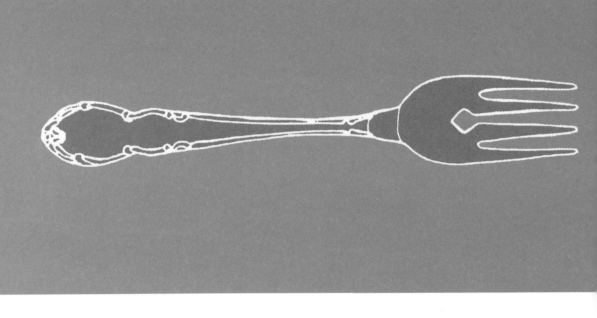

COLLARD GREENS

Collard greens, a deep green, slightly bitter member of the cabbage family, have been cultivated for millennia. Some more modern ways to cook them up:

→ Chop the greens and slowly simmer in salted vegetable stock with a dash of liquid smoke or chipotle peppers until soft.

→ Use raw or lightly steamed collard greens as a wrap, instead of using a tortilla or nori sheet.

→ Spread peanut or almond butter on a collard leaf and roll it up for a healthful snack.

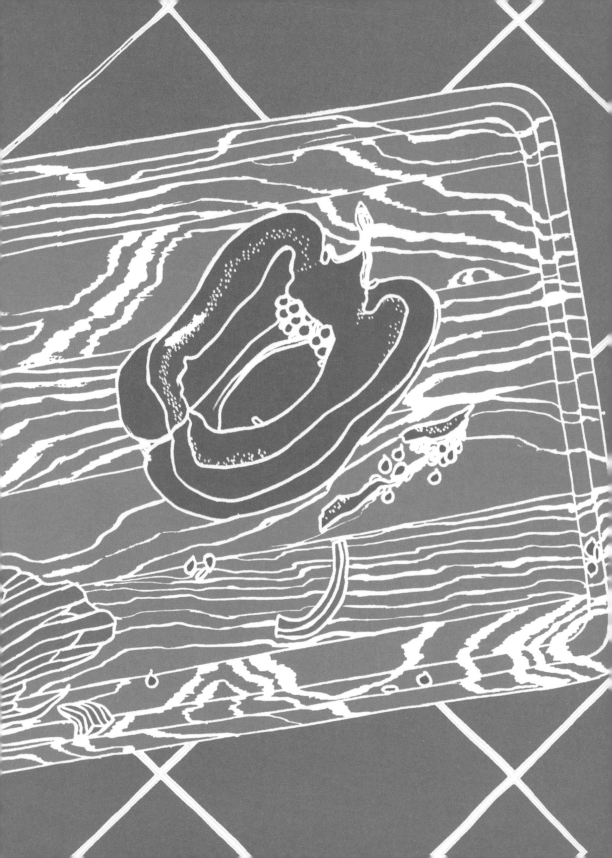

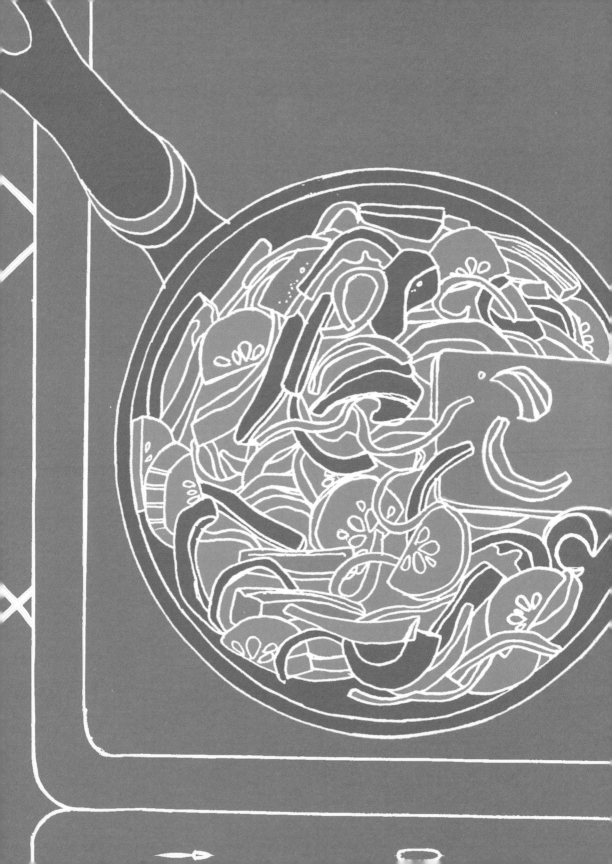

VOLUNTEER

Many vegans want to be actively involved in helping animals but often struggle with what role we can play. The bottom line is that you will be most effective at something you are good at and enjoy. In reflecting upon your skills and interests, what can you contribute to animal rights organizations you admire? What are your answers to: What am I good at? What need can I fill?

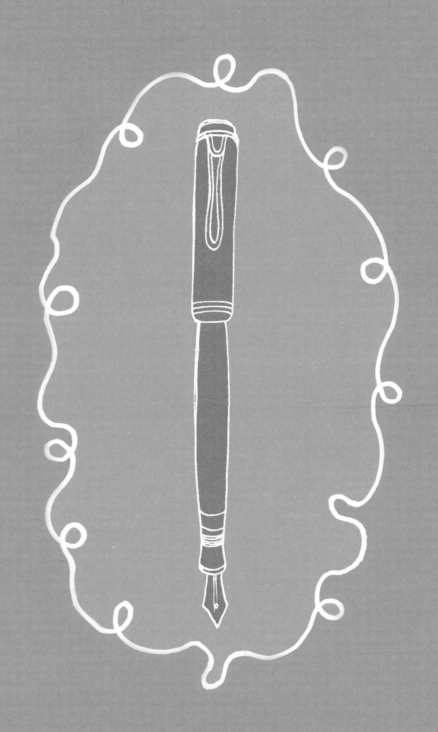

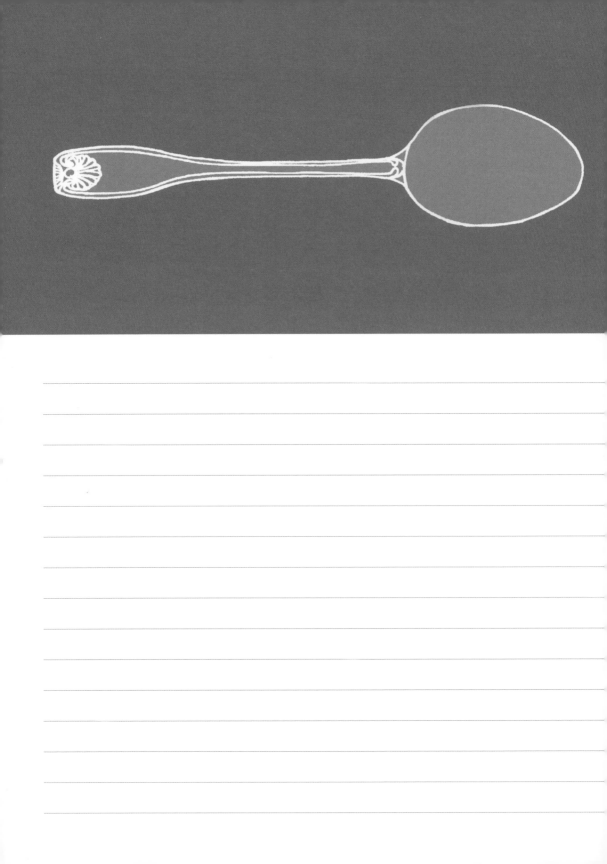

OLIVES

The olive in its natural state is not edible. Before you buy them, they are soaked and cured to remove bitter flavors. Look for brine-cured, water-cured or dry-salted olives. There are dozens to try—from small, firm, meaty Manzanilla olives, often stuffed with garlic or pimento; to deep-purple Kalamata olives, which are great in salads and sauces; and rich, nutty Nicoise olives, which are a tempting pre-meal snack.

Do they know, as we do, that their time must come?

Yes, they know, at rare moments.

No other way can I interpret those pauses of his latter life, when, propped on his forefe
he would sit for long minutes quite motionless—
His head drooped, utterly withdrawn; then turn those eyes of his and look at me.

That look said more plainly than all words could:
"Yes, I know that I must go."
If we have spirits that persist—they have.

— From "Do They Know?" by John Galsworthy

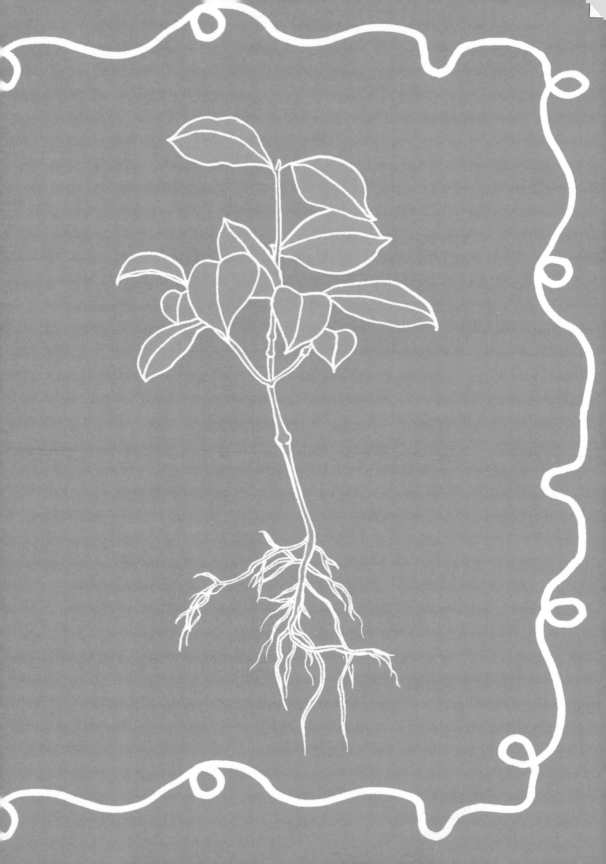

First published in the United States of America in 2015 by
Quarry Books, a member of
Quarto Publishing Group USA Inc.
100 Cummings Center
Suite 406-L
Beverly, Massachusetts 01915-6101
Telephone: (978) 282-9590
Fax: (978) 283-2742
www.quarrybooks.com
Visit www.QuarrySPOON.com and help us celebrate food and culture one spoonful at a time!

10 9 8 7 6 5 4 3 2 1

ISBN: 978-1-63159-006-1

Design: Leigh Ring // www.ringartdesign.com
Cover Image: Leigh Ring // www.ringartdesign.com
Illustrations: Dayna Safferstein

Printed in China